The Make-Up Book

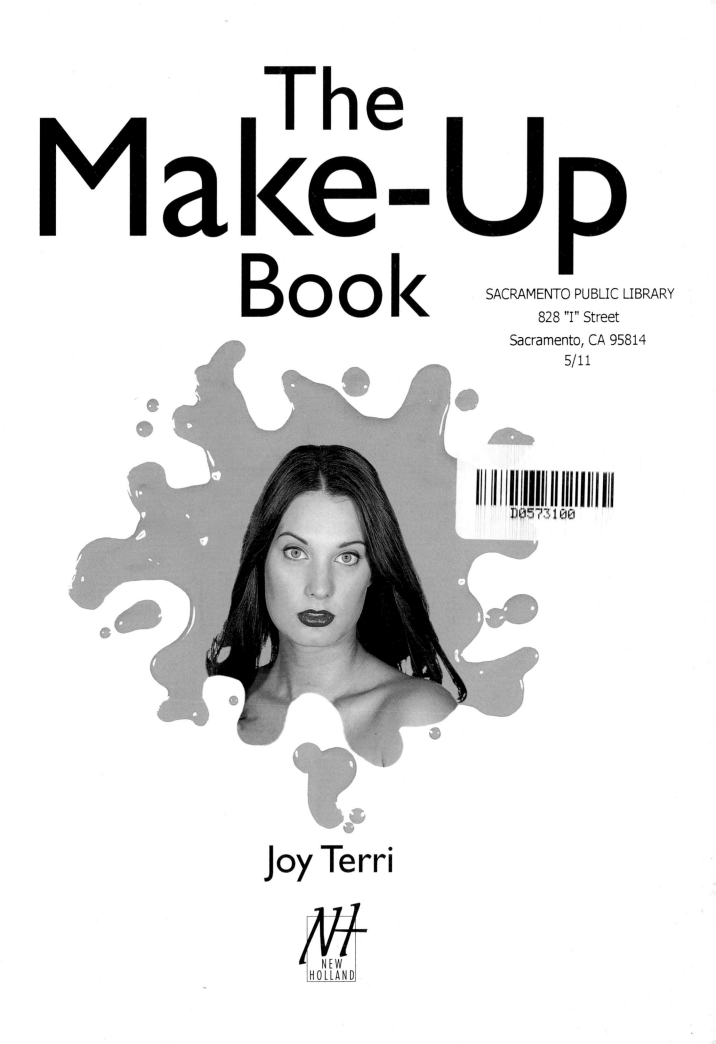

Joy Terri

NH
NEW
HOLLAND

This paperback edition published in 2011

First published in 1999 by New Holland Publishers (UK) Ltd

London • Cape Town • Sydney • Auckland

10 9 8 7 6 5 4 3 2 1

Garfield House, 86-88 Edgware Road
London, W2 2EA
United Kingdom

80 McKenzie Street
Cape Town 8001
South Africa

Unit 1, 66 Gibbes Street
Chatswood, NSW 2067
Australia

218 Lake Road
Northcote, Auckland
New Zealand

Publishing director: Linda de Villiers
Editor: Laura Milton
Design director: Janice Evans
Designer: Beverley Dodd
Make-up and styling: Joy Terri
Hairstylist: Donald Olive
Illustrator: Alix Korte

All photographs taken by Sean Waller, with the exception of the following: cover front (bottom, far right), pages 28 (bottom right), 39 (bottom left and right), 46 (bottom right), 67 (bottom left and right), 89 (second from the bottom), 91, 92 (bottom left and right), 93 (top left and right) and 94 (bottom left and right) by Henry Martin; and pages 3 (third from the bottom), 6, 58 (bottom left), 67 (top), 87 (top row and bottom right) and 88 by Kelly Walsh.

Reproduction by Hirt & Carter Cape (Pty) Ltd
Printed and bound In Malaysia by Times Offset (M) Sdn Bhd

ISBN 978 1 84773 932 2

author's acknowledgements

Very special thanks to my best friend and business partner, Debbie Jean, whose initial idea it was for me to write the book, and who motivated and supported me through it.

Thank you to my two very special make-up artists, Kerry Williams and Debbie Collins. Not only did you both give me moral support throughout working on the book, but also endless days of hard work. Your talents as make-up artists and models helped make this book possible.

An enormous thank you to Donald and the team at Sloanes Hair Company (especially Donovan) for your work on the hair in this book. Your excellent work motivated and assisted me and I couldn't have done it without you. I cannot think of better people to work with.

Thank you Sean Waller for the excellent photography. It was a great pleasure to work with you. Also thanks to both Kelly Walsh and Henry Martin for their photography.

And thank you, Alix, for your beautiful illustrations.

A special thank you to my editor, Laura, for your care, attention to detail and complete involvement in this book. I hope that we will be able to work together again in the future.

And special thanks to my designer, Bev, for your inspirational work that has made this book into what I wished it to be.

Thanks also to Linda and everyone else at Struik involved with producing this book.

I would also like to thank those who gave up their time to model for various sections in the book: Abeeda, Alayne, Alindi, Denise, Karen, Janice, Joanna, Jean, June, Lia, Lindy, Leander, Mom, Melanie, Sandy, Sibongele, Ying-Hung. Also, for your time, thanks to Wendy and Lindy W, Rosaline, Kim and Elanor.

Special thanks to André for all your love and patience. I couldn't have wished for better help and support during this time.

Thank you Duran and Rayne for your sacrifices throughout this book.

Thank you Mom and Dad for the love and support, as well as the enthusiasm you've shown for every project I've worked on. I thank you for where I am today and I hope to show my appreciation through making you as proud of me as I am of you.

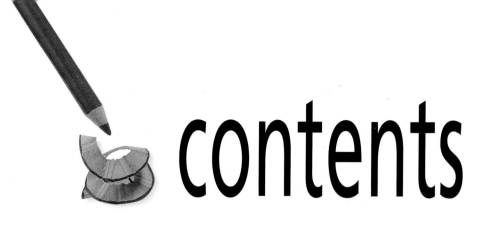

contents

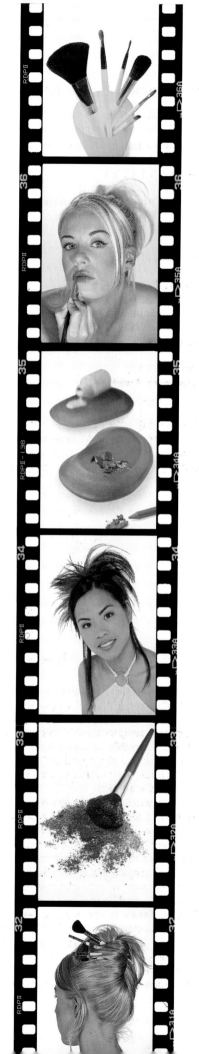

introduction

For years the art of applying make-up has been regarded as something mysterious taking place 'behind the scenes' in the fashion and film industry, with the magical 'tricks of the trade' applied to models and film stars only. The truth is that, with professional guidance, every woman can learn to use make-up to make the most of herself. In this book I would like to introduce some of the specialist products, tools and techniques that are at your disposal to help you create the exact effect you desire.

Make-up trends, like fashions in clothing, undergo constant change. Certain colours periodically gain popularity, as do certain styles. We are each offered a unique opportunity to respond – whether we accept, adapt or reject. Although many women will readily update their wardrobes to include something of the latest season's colours and styles, they are less likely to adapt their make-up to keep pace with changing trends and the development of new products. Some women only ever learn one way of applying make-up to their faces, and never stop to question what they are doing.

Women who 'decorate' their faces without questioning their technique often become so used to the 'decoration' that they begin relying on this look. They seldom, if ever, seek professional advice and never discover their true potential. If they do seek advice, they usually speak to a saleslady at a cosmetics counter who may also lack professional knowledge, and who may agree to almost anything that will help her sell her products.

Applied correctly, make-up can enhance a woman's beauty by accentuating striking features, or creating visual illusions, for example. A woman can use make-up to help her project an image of natural beauty, elegance or power, depending on what is appropriate. Applied incorrectly, however, make-up can actually detract from a woman's looks. A face may look different after make-up has been applied, but not necessarily better. A 'plain' face may merely be turned into a 'decorated' face, instead of a fresh-looking, elegant, or more youthful face.

Have you ever asked yourself whether you would allow anyone but a professional hairstylist to cut your hair? I do not not know any woman who would happily sport a noticeably 'amateur' haircut. When it comes to applying make-up, though, most women never consider that they may be creating a clearly 'amateur' look, and may even have been creating the same one for years.

The explanation may lie in the fact that make-up is so easy to remove. Imagine how much care we would take if we knew that, once applied, our make-up would be permanent, or even semi-permanent.

Not only do I love my work as a professional make-up artist, but I have also learned to make the most of my own looks. The self-confidence I have gained has made me a much happier, more positive and successful person, and I am passionate about sharing my knowledge with other women.

Everything you need to know has been brought together in this book, but, as in the case of any practical subject, you need to dedicate some time to learning the 'theory' and some time to practising the techniques described.

If you apply make-up at all, you will probably be applying it to your face for the rest of your life, so some hours spent practising now will prove to be a sound investment in your future.

As I said earlier, make-up trends change over the years, but the key to always looking your best lies in possessing knowledge of the winning combination of the correct make-up products, tools and professional techniques. Once you have gained this knowledge and mastered the various techniques, you will always be able to adapt your make-up look to being fashionable, whilst at the same time enhancing your particular features and making the most of your unique looks.

Joy Terri

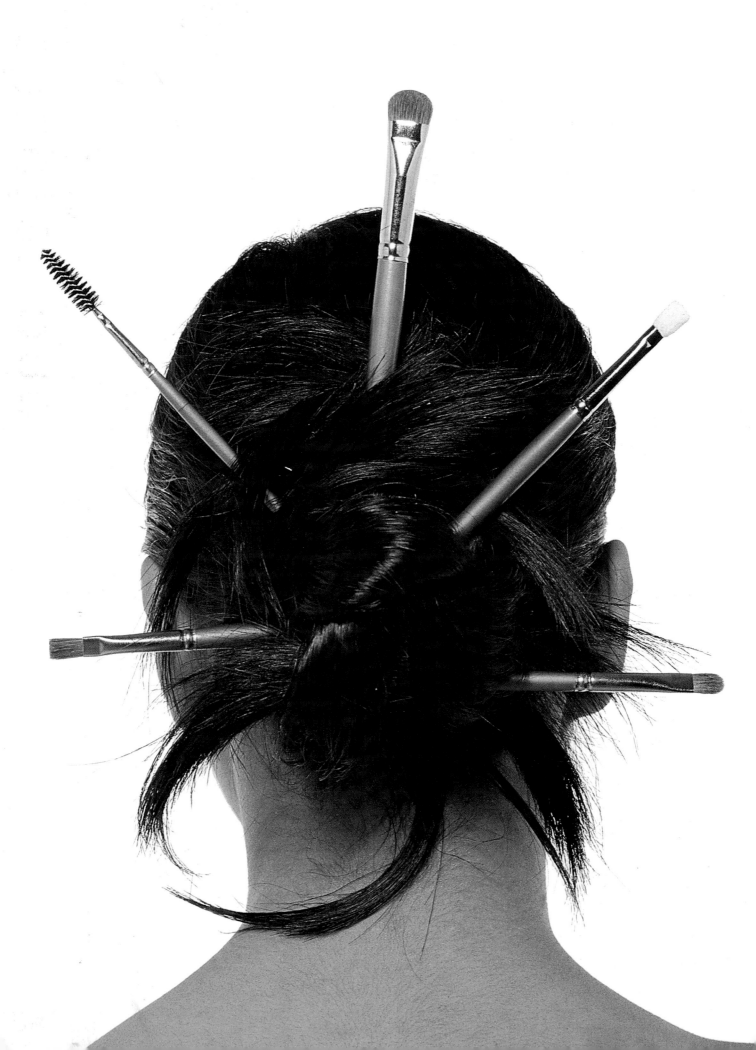

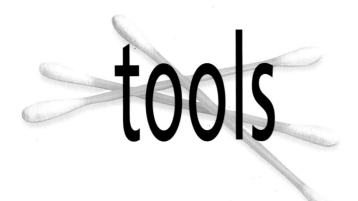

tools

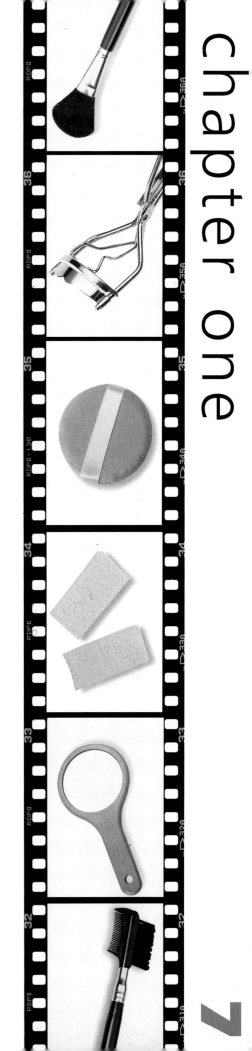

Quality make-up tools are an excellent investment – not meant only for use by professionals. If you are serious about looking your best at all times, and you are investing time in learning how experts in the field set to work, you also need to acquire the correct equipment. This chapter will show you what you need.

tools
of the trade

Many women will spend a fortune on make-up products, only to use inferior tools when it comes to applying those products to the skin. Avoid this costly mistake – pay as much attention to the applicator as to the product. It is no good using an excellent product, but botching the application because you lack the appropriate applicator. Once this is understood, it will be clear why I begin this book by addressing the choice of make-up tools.

Obtaining the correct applicators may seem like a daunting task at first, but, believe me, you will soon realize what a difference the right tools can make. Your make-up application will become quicker and easier, and the results you achieve will be far more professional. And although a good make-up brush may seem quite expensive initially, remember that, with care, it could last a lifetime. Whilst make-up products date, run out or break into pieces, professional make-up tools are never wasted. Don't skimp – you will find that having more make-up tools means that you need fewer, possibly more versatile, products. Use a separate brush for each colour or product you apply, otherwise successful blending becomes almost impossible.

If possible, buy your tools from a professional make-up supplier. This will ensure quality, and save you from wasting money on expensive gimmicks. If you live far from a major centre, find out whether your nearest professional supplier is willing to mail your order to you (see page 95). All of the tools discussed on the pages that follow are available from professional make-up suppliers, and many of them are stocked by good department stores, pharmacies or health shops.

I recommend the following basic tools and accessories for your personal make-up kit.

general tools

a small sea sponge

A natural sea sponge, harvested when small, is soft and unabrasive. It is used for applying liquid foundation. Once wet, it has the advantage of not wasting the foundation by absorbing as much of it as a synthetic sponge would.

Wet the sponge thoroughly, squeeze out the water, then squeeze the sponge once more between the layers of a towel or in a tissue before using it to apply your foundation. Rinse it immediately after use.

latex sponges

These sponges are extremely handy, as they can be used for various purposes, for example:

- ◆ in conjunction with a sea sponge to blend away edges or streaks of liquid foundation
- ◆ to apply powder or cream foundations
- ◆ to blend concealer.

Although latex sponges are available in different shapes and forms, the wedge shape is ideal for blending close to the eyelashes, as well as into the creases around the nostrils.

I prefer to work with these sponges when they are dry, but some make-up artists prefer to dampen the sponges first. Wash sponges once a week to keep them unclogged and free from grime, and replace a wedge as soon as it begins breaking up or changing texture.

powder puff

Use this puff to press powder onto your face. This procedure is the key to 'setting' your make-up. If you have been using a brush up until now, try a puff instead. You will notice a marked difference in terms of how long your make-up lasts, as a brush does not set the foundation in the same way as is done by using a patting action and a puff.

Good powder puffs are stitched together at the seams, not glued. They can easily be washed without coming apart.

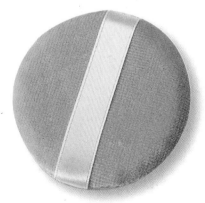

eyelash curler

This is a wonderful tool for those of us not blessed with lashes with a natural curl. It is not suggested that you use a curler every day – save it for special occasions.

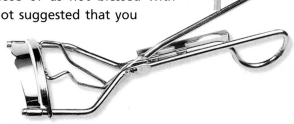

tweezer

This is an essential tool for removing hair and maintaining a good eyebrow shape. Although tweezers are generally quite easy to find, it is worthwhile spending some time ensuring you find some that grip the hair really well. You may have to try out various brands.

sharpener

Sharp pencils are a must – for lips, eyes and brows. Invest in a versatile sharpener of good quality, and keep it clean.

handbag-sized shopping mirror

It is always a good idea to have this at the ready whenever you are shopping for make-up. It is next to impossible to test product colours inside stores using artificial light. If you have your own small mirror, you can walk to a source of natural light in the store and inspect the product you are testing on your face there. Make sure that your mirror is not too small – the mirrored section should not be smaller than the palm of your hand.

cotton buds & tissues

These disposable and inexpensive items come in handy at many different stages of make-up application. Cotton buds are ideal for blending make-up around the eye, and tissues are used to blot lipstick as well as to dust excess make-up off brushes during the process of application.

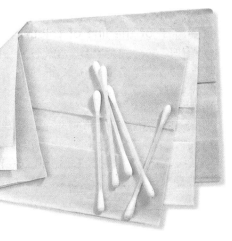

make-up brushes

powder brush

Use the largest brush in your kit as your powder brush. It should be soft and very smooth to the touch. First apply powder using a puff (see page 9), and then use this large brush to dust the excess powder from your face.

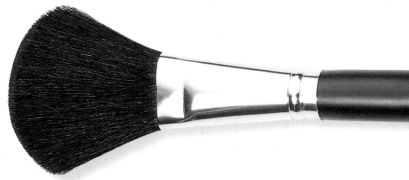

blusher brush

The best brush for applying blusher is more or less the size of the one pictured on the right. In addition to providing natural, healthy-looking colour, blusher is usually used to define the cheekbone and contour the face. If you use a larger

brush, the blusher tends to colour too large an area of the cheek, or it creates an unflattering and obvious wide 'band' of colour. Using the correct brush will enable you to apply the colour far more precisely – both in terms of the amount of colour applied, as well as its position. Select a brush in which the brush hairs are not all cut to one length, but graduate gently, with shorter hairs on the outsides and longer hair at the centre. This will ensure an even distribution of blusher across the cheek, and help you avoid a 'patchy' look.

blusher blending brush

Your blending brush can be larger than your blusher brush and the hair can either be graduated or cut to one length. After applying blusher, the 'edges' of the line of colour are often too obvious, and so you need a clean brush to blend and soften the shape of the coloured area. This brush should never be dipped into the container of your blusher so that it becomes coated with blusher itself. It should always be kept clean and only be used for blending.

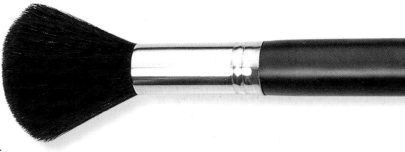

dome-shaped eye-shadow brushes

Small, dome-shaped brushes are used for applying eye shadows. A separate brush must be used for each colour of shadow used, for instance one for shading and one for highlighting. In brushes of this shape, the hair is graduated from short to long in a rounded, dome shape. As the hairs do not end in a straight line, the particles of eye-shadow powder cling to the brush evenly along the shaped part.

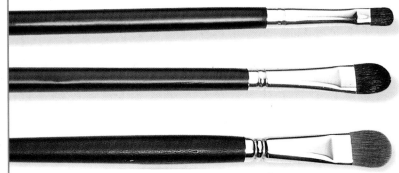

When the brush touches the skin, therefore, the powder is not all deposited in one patch. The brush allows the particles of shadow to be distributed evenly across the eyelid.

Dome-shaped brushes are available in different sizes. Larger brushes are used to shade larger areas on the eye, and smaller brushes for smaller areas. The best small brushes are made of sable hair – this is smooth and soft, and does not pull or tug at the skin in the delicate eye area. Your smallest brush should be soft, yet firm enough to enable you to apply eye shadow close to the upper and lower lashes in a neat, thin line. This is useful when lining the eyes with dark eye shadow (see page 69), rather than using pencil eyeliner.

flat eye-shadow brush

This flat brush with the hair tips ending in a straight line is used to blend away hard edges of eye-shadow colour. As is the case with a brush used to blend blusher, this brush should not be dipped into the powder container at all, but be kept clean and used only for blending away hard lines.

These brushes are not the most effective when applying powder or eye shadow. As mentioned previously, the powder particles collect along the end of the hair in a straight line and, when applied to the skin, there is not a gradual distribution of colour. Often a 'blotch' of shadow is deposited where all the powder lands as the brush touches the skin.

Straight-edged, flat brushes should never be 'dipped' into eye shadow or blusher in a container (see page 64). They tend to hit the product with more force than a dome-shaped brush. This often leads to compacted powder products breaking up into pieces, and much of the product thus being wasted.

liquid eyeliner brush

If you use liquid eyeliner often, it is worthwhile investing in one of these brushes. It makes the application so much easier. This professional brush designed specifically for lining eyes is made of sable hair which graduates towards a clean point. You

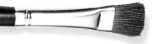

will be able to apply a clean, neat line, without the hair separating.

eyebrow brush, eyelash comb & mascara wand

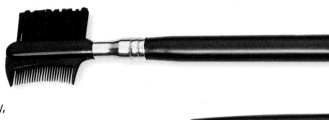

The little brush shown here is used to brush eyebrows up and outwards to create a neat shape. Apply mascara using the appropriate wand and, if necessary, use the small comb to comb the mascara through the lashes evenly, removing any 'blobs'. Many make-up artists also use a wand-type applicator for brushing eyebrows effectively.

angled eyebrow brush

This is used instead of or with an eyebrow pencil to apply shadow to the eyebrows, to darken them or to fill in spaces created by uneven hair growth. The slanted shape is ideal for creating the illusion of small, slanting eyebrow hairs in between existing ones.

The brush shown here is made of hog hair, but similar brushes are available made from sable hair. If your eyebrow hair is fine, choose sable hair; if your eyebrow hair is coarse, choose a brush made of hog hair.

lipstick brush

As lipstick is such a sticky substance, a firm brush is required for its successful application. Brushes made of sable hair are generally best for working the lipstick onto your lips. Some make-up artists prefer working with quite small lipstick brushes to ensure a clean lip edge, however, as clean an edge can be achieved using an average-sized brush carefully.

concealer brush

Concealer is also a sticky substance like lipstick, so once again a small sable hair brush is ideal. For concealing blemishes, a brush with a very fine tip is necessary so that only a tiny dot of concealer can be applied at a time. The aim is to cover the blemish alone – not the surrounding area.

fan brush

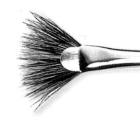

This brush is an optional extra, used for dusting off loose powder. Its shape is ideal for sweeping excess powder away from the eye area. It can also reach into the creases at the sides of the nose.

natural or synthetic hair?

Manufacturers of make-up brushes have realized that women often purchase brushes or commercial brush kits because they look colourful and attractive, rather than because of their particular shape, size or texture. This has meant that simple, good make-up brushes have become quite hard to find. Colourful brushes in pretty pots that match the colour scheme of your bedroom may look nice, but often very little thought has gone into the real purpose of the brushes.

Cheap, colourful brushes are often made using synthetic hair, which is coarse and scratchy. These brushes damage make-up products in compacted powder form, as they quickly break them up into dust, and the brush hairs have rarely been cut into the correct domed shape to apply make-up successfully. The hair of synthetic brushes also often loses its shape quite soon. The brush too easily flares into a 'fountain' shape, making application rather difficult and messy.

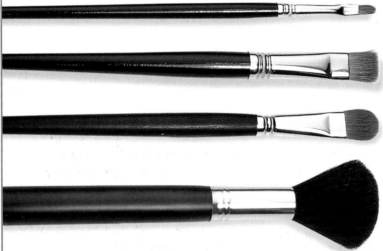

Professional make-up brushes are made of natural animal hair. Depending on the flexibility requirements of the brush, a particular choice of hair is made. For eye-shadow brushes, sable hair is the most suitable, although it may also be the most expensive. Sable hair is soft, smooth and gentle on the delicate skin around the eye. At the same time, it has the correct degree of firmness required for effective make-up application. Brushes for applying blusher and powder are made of softer natural hair.

Professional brushes made of natural hair are also very carefully cut into shapes designed for particular purposes. Make-up application becomes neater, easier and quicker. In addition, used correctly, brushes made of natural hair do not damage compact eye shadows and blushers as much as synthetic brushes, so you will find that your make-up products last far longer.

Brushes made of natural hair may seem expensive initially, but they are made to last. They save you constantly having to replace brushes, or products that have been broken into bits by coarse and scratchy synthetic brushes.

cleaning your brushes

All your make-up brushes should be cleaned at least once a month. Brushes used to apply lipstick and concealer require more frequent cleaning than brushes used for powder products, though, as these brushes often become sticky and then easily pick up particles of dust and dirt.

Brushes can be washed in warm water with pure soap or mild hair shampoo. Make sure that you wash brushes gently, retaining the shape of the brush hair and not flaring it out into a fountain shape. Gently squeeze out the make-up while the brush is under the water. Follow the same procedure and rinse brushes thoroughly in clean water, ensuring that all traces of soapiness have been removed. Squeeze the hair back into its original shape and place the brushes on a clean, dry towel to dry.

Make-up brushes may also be cleaned without water, just by using certain quite strong chemicals. Until recently these chemicals have only been available professionally, owing to their toxicity and danger in the home environment. Some manufacturers have now come up with non-toxic formulas, though, and these can be ordered from professional make-up suppliers. You simply dip your brushes into the cleaner, remove them and wipe them on a tissue. They are dry almost immediately, as the cleaner evaporates instantly. It only takes seconds to completely remove even sticky red lipstick from your brush.

space & light

It is important to create a comfortable space for everyday make-up application. There is no point investing in tools and products, and learning professional techniques if you are going to try to apply your make-up using the rear-view mirror of your car on your way to work every day, for example.

Firstly, you need sufficient space to set out your make-up kit in front of you. As make-up containers are generally difficult to keep clean, it may be a good idea to get into the habit of unpacking all the products you need, and opening all the lids before you begin applying anything. When you have completed your application, wash or wipe your fingers, close all the containers, and return them to your make-up bag. You will find that the containers and the bag stay remarkably clean.

When applying make-up, it is essential that light is distributed evenly over your face. Always use a cool lamp, and one that emits light which is as close as possible in colour to natural daylight. Normal household globes emit considerable heat and create a yellow glow that can be quite misleading when you select make-up colours.

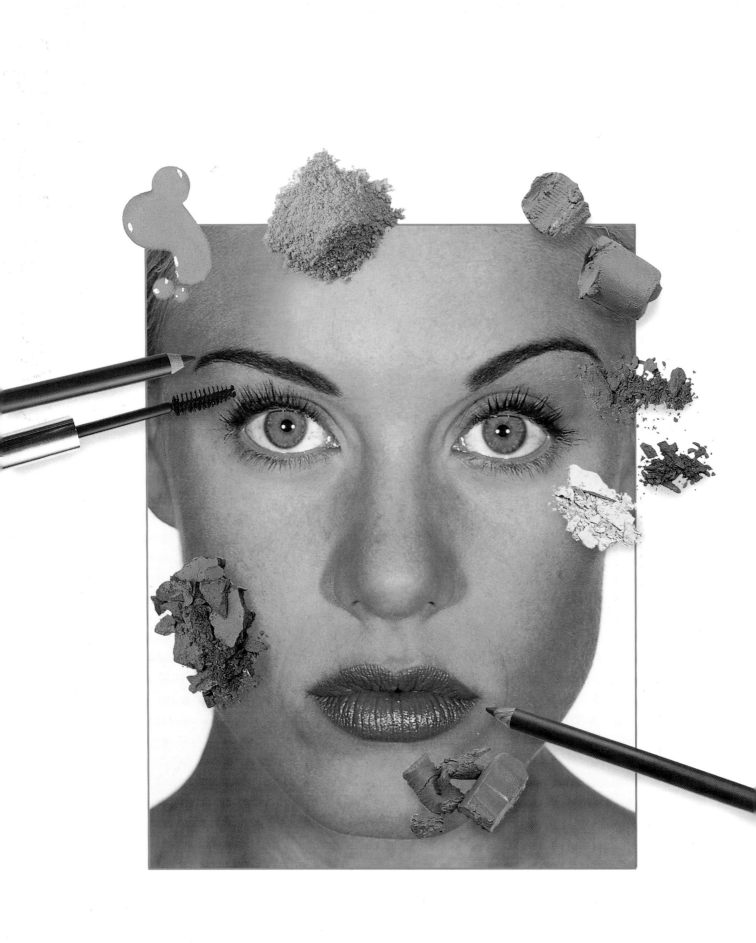

products

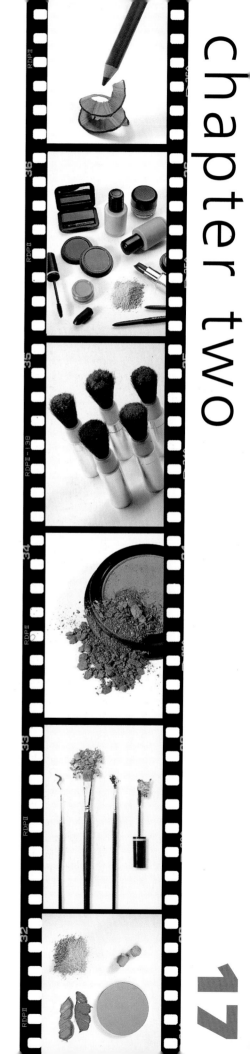

To achieve a truly professional make-up finish you not only require the correct tools, but also the correct make-up products. So as not to be overwhelmed by the array of products facing you, it is essential to have a clear understanding of the functions of each product.

basic
explanations

In my view it is of great importance to have a clear understanding the function of each make-up product used during the application process. This will enable you to identify exactly what you need, and to shop accordingly. You will also know what the specific product should be able to accomplish for you, and what you can and cannot expect from it. Testers at make-up counters not only allow you to test the *colour* of a product on your skin, but also to judge its *quality and texture* in terms of the particular function you require it to perform.

There should, for example, be a distinct difference in texture between a pencil used for eyebrows, and one used as an eyeliner. Knowing what to look for – and not simply reading the manufacturer's label on the pencil – is what counts. The same goes for other make-up products and, if you are not satisfied with what you find in the shops, you can always contact a professional make-up supplier (see page 95).

This chapter gives an overview of the basic products used to put together a good make-up kit. Once you have a good grasp of the function of each product, and are aware of what is available, you will be able to make an informed choice about which type of product you require.

foundation

Foundation products are used to create an even skin tone, and to smooth the skin texture to create a seemingly flawless finish. Foundation is meant to provide light to medium coverage, not to cover pigmentation marks, blemishes, dark rings under the eyes and so forth – this is why you may require a separate concealer.

Foundation also provides a base for the subsequent application of other make-up products Eye shadows, blushers and lipsticks, for instance, are not designed for use on skin without foundation. In fact, if you add colours to the 'naked' face without using foundation, the make-up colour you add will exaggerate the unevenness in the skin tone and could result in blemishes and flaws being more noticeable. In addition, other products will not blend or last as well on skin without foundation.

Quite possibly nothing is more important than finding (or mixing) foundation to match your skin colour exactly. A 'close' match is simply not good enough – it has to be exact and 'invisible' once applied.

Nowadays a vast range of foundation products is available. Textures vary enormously, in addition to being water-based, oil-based or oil-free, and consistency and coverage differ greatly. Most good make-up houses offer a wide range of colours to match your skin tone. Take time to experiment – it is your right be assertive and to insist on testing and comparing various brands. Foundation usually takes one of three basic forms: liquid, cream, or powder.

liquid foundation

Liquids generally offer light to medium coverage, but the precise extent of coverage depends on the particular brand and on how thickly the liquid is applied.

Liquid foundations offer the widest range of colours, and if you are unable to find an exact match to your skin tone, colours can be mixed to obtain an in-between shade. Do not mix foundations of different brands, though. Keep to products of the same kind from a single make-up house. If you have never used foundation, there is no need to be concerned that your face will look unnaturally 'painted'. If foundation is matched to the skin tone exactly, a wonderfully natural appearance can be achieved.

For very dry skin, choose an oil-based foundation. For normal skin, choose a water-based foundation, and for very oily skin, choose foundation labelled 'oil-free'.

cream foundation

A cream that feels slightly dry to the touch will usually offer light to medium cover. Very rich, often stodgy creams offer medium to heavy cover, and are used mostly for stage and film make-up. These heavier creams are not suggested for use on mature skin.

powder foundation

This type of foundation was developed more recently than liquid or cream foundations. It has been designed for women who need to apply their make-up in a hurry or for those who dislike the feel of liquid or cream foundation on the skin.

Powder foundation can be understood as two products combined into one – foundation and powder. When using other types of foundation, the subsequent application of powder is required to 'set' the foundation. If you use a powder foundation, however, you can omit a separate, subsequent application of powder.

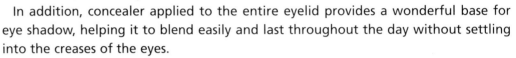

concealer

This product is applied to provide extra cover to specific areas where foundation has not been sufficient to create an even skin tone. It may be used to conceal blemishes, dark rings under the eyes, or unwanted redness still obvious on the cheeks, nose or chin, for example.

In addition, concealer applied to the entire eyelid provides a wonderful base for eye shadow, helping it to blend easily and last throughout the day without settling into the creases of the eyes.

It is important that your concealer is one or two shades lighter in colour than your foundation, but that it has the same undertone. For example, if your foundation is beige with a yellowish undertone, then your concealer should also have a yellowish undertone, and not a pinkish one.

Concealer is available in several forms: mainly as a liquid, as a stick, and as a cream.

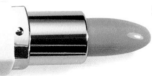

liquid concealer

The packaging of this form of concealer often contains a wand applicator. The advantage of a liquid is that it blends softly and easily without you having to tug at the skin. While being useful for concealing pigmentation on the eyelids, for instance, this kind of concealer does not offer enough cover to mask blemishes.

stick concealer

This form of concealer generally offers good cover for blemishes. It may be difficult to blend without pulling the skin, however, so avoid using it around the delicate eye area.

cream concealer

This concealer, often packaged in a small tub, is the form of concealer most commonly used by make-up artists because it has the perfect consistency. Cream concealers have the advantages of both the liquid and stick forms, without any of the disadvantages. The cream is sticky enough to cling to areas that require cover, while also being soft enough to blend easily. It is good for concealing blemishes, dark rings under the eyes, or undesirable red tinges still showing through the foundation. It is also soft and comfortable enough to use around the eye area without stretching the skin during application.

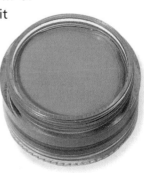

powder

There are several very good reasons for using powder. Most importantly, powder 'sets' your foundation and makes it last. It also adds a matte finish that always looks fresh, professional, and chic. Powder can make the skin texture seem finer, as it makes the pores look smaller. Lastly, powder removes any stickiness created by foundation or concealer. After powdering, eye shadow or blusher can be applied and blended easily on a silky smooth skin.

It is very important to ensure that the powder you use does not change the colour of your foundation. If you have succeeded in matching your foundation to your skin colour perfectly, you do not want to change it now by applying powder that contains too much colour, especially not pink.

Powder is generally available in loose, translucent form or in pressed form.

loose, translucent powder

Most of the loose powders offered by make-up houses are not translucent in the true sense of the word, as they inevitably contain a certain amount of colour. In addition, there are usually only a few shades to choose from. Therefore, most make-up artists prefer using professional translucent powder that does not contain any real colouring. By so doing they do not risk changing the foundation colour already carefully matched to the skin.

Loose powder does not build up on the skin and create a heavy, caked look. It is extremely light and if too much is applied, the excess can easily be dusted off with a large, soft brush.

pressed powder

The one distinct advantage of pressed powder is that it is much less messy to carry in your handbag than loose powder. For this reason, it can sometimes be handy for quick touch-ups during the course of the day. You also generally have a wider range of shades to choose from than in the case of loose powder. If you opt for pressed powder, find a shade as close as possible to the colour of your foundation, and only use it sparingly. The disadvantage of pressed powder is that it tends to build up on the skin if applied repeatedly, and one needs to be aware of this when doing touch-ups.

yellow colour correctors

The majority of women have yellowy skin tones, rather than pink skin tones. Make-up houses have overlooked this fact for years, and many of them have been manufacturing foundations, concealers and powders containing far too much pink colouring for their make-up products to look completely natural. The aim of foundations, concealers and powders is to make skin seem flawless. If the products applied differ from the natural skin colour, though, a really natural look with 'invisible' make-up cannot be achieved.

Some make-up houses have begun to realize that they need to improve their colour ranges, and they are beginning to produce products with yellower tones, as well as yellow colour correctors to be mixed with their other products. If these correctors are not yet freely available in your part of the world, contact a professional make-up supplier (see page 95) and you may arrange a mail order.

Yellow powder is a translucent powder with an added yellow colouring. It can be used to create a finish as close as possible to one's natural skin tone. As a make-up artist, I use yellow powder on women with all skin tones, with the exception of those who are very fair.

To match certain skin tones I find that, in addition to using yellow powder, I also need to add a yellow base to the foundation to achieve a perfect match. Add as little or as much corrector as you need to match your skin.

eyebrow pencil

This kind of pencil is used to define and darken the eyebrows, or to pencil them in, and to create the illusion of even hair growth throughout the length of the brow. A good eyebrow pencil needs to be hard and dry, so that you can draw crisp, clean lines, and not create smudgy brows that look painted. Many pencils that are labelled 'eyebrow pencil' are far too soft to create the desired effect. Before buying, test the texture of the pencil by drawing on the back of your hand – the line should be crisp.

In terms of colour, eyebrow pencils are generally available in black, dark brown, light brown and grey. If you choose a light brown colour, take care not to choose one with a strong rusty tinge to it – this colour almost always looks 'false' unless you are a true fiery redhead. If you are very fair, it is safest to choose a pale ash-brown colour.

eyebrow shadow

This is used instead of pencil or sometimes applied over eyebrow pencil to create a natural finish. It can only be used as a pencil substitute where there is substantial hair growth. In fact, many make-up artists actually prefer using shadow to pencil in the latter case. Eyebrow shadow alone should not be used where hair growth is very sparse.

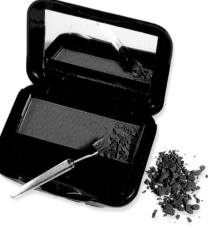

eye shadow

Make-up in the form of eye shadow is used around the eyes to draw attention to them and to enhance their natural shape. Eye shadow is available in pressed and loose powder forms, as well as in cream forms, and in matte, frosted or iridescent formulas. It is probably most widely available in pressed powder form, and the range of colours and shades is vast. On pages 48–57 colours have been categorized to guide you in selecting which are suitable.

As a general rule I recommend that you have three shades of eye shadow to work with during a single application:

- a light colour (white, for example), referred to as your *highlighter*
- a medium or darkish shade (medium brown, for example), referred to as your *shading colour*
- a very dark shade (dark brown/black, for example), referred to as your *framing colour*.

eyeliner

This is used to create a darkened frame around each eye, drawing attention to the eyes and accentuating their beauty. Eyeliner can also be used to create illusions around the eyes, making them appear larger, or more elongated, for example.

It is very important that you always choose pencil eyeliners that are very soft, so that shading can gently and easily be applied to the delicate skin around the eye. Pencils used on this area should not scratch or tug at the skin, thereby stretching it. The shading should blend easily if you want to soften the line with a cotton bud. Test pencils before buying by drawing on your hand and then smudging the line gently. Pencil eyeliners are available in assorted colours, but for equipping an everyday make-up kit I recommend dark brown and/or black.

Not only pencils are used to outline eyes, though, as many make-up artists prefer using very dark eye shadow. Some never use a pencil at all, because shadow is softer on the skin and looks more natural than a hard, pencilled line. The quality of eye shadow used is important, though, as you should be able to apply it neatly without messing. Shadow will also last longer around the eye than pencil.

I do not recommend liquid eyeliner for everyday use, as it can so easily look messy if not applied correctly. I have therefore discussed it separately on page 25.

mascara

This is used to thicken and darken the eyelashes which, in turn, enhance the beauty of the eyes. Mascara is generally available in dark brown, black and charcoal grey, as well as in various consistencies in regular and waterproof formulas. Although it is also available in navy, blue, and a number of other colours, these are fashion fads. Do not make a habit of using them regularly. And remember, if you use waterproof mascara, you will need an appropriate remover.

blusher

The function of blusher is either to define the cheekbone or to soften a cheekbone that is too prominent, and to enhance and contour the shape of the face. Blusher can also be used to add natural colour to the face. These aspects are discussed in detail on pages 74–77.

Blushers are available in pressed powder and cream forms. Whichever form you choose, keep to natural colours with a matte finish. Never choose a bright pink or a bright orange blusher. This will defeat the purpose of the application.

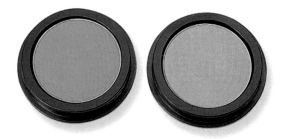

lip pencil

Lips are outlined to define the mouth and create a clean, neat border for lipstick application. Lip liners can also be used to correct the shape of the lips if they are unbalanced, for instance, by enlarging a top lip slightly. This is much easier to accomplish when using a lip pencil than it is when using lipstick alone (see pages 81–83).

When choosing a lip pencil, test the quality on the back of your hand. It should not be soft and smudgy. Lip pencils are made with less oil and from a much harder wax than lipstick. This is done so that your lip outline will last, and not 'bleed' beyond the lip edge the way lipstick can. Lip liners are available in a variety of colours and should be matched as closely as possible to your lipstick colour.

lipstick

A neat application of a suitable lipstick adds finish to a look and colour to the face. In addition, it draws attention to your lips, and to your smile. Most lipsticks sold at cosmetics counters are presented in a stick form. Lipsticks are available in cream and frosted formulas, and in a wide variety of colours. Some offer a high degree of coverage and the appearance of solid colour, while others are more sheer, working with the natural lip colour. Some formulas have been designed to last through several hours of wear without requiring reapplication. When buying lipstick, test various colours and textures, as some may feel very dry on the lips. Then choose the formula you find most comfortable to wear.

optional extras

As technology develops, new or improved 'problem-solving' products are constantly appearing on the shelves. These are not essentials, but can be exceptionally useful.

anti-shine

This is a great product for applying to oily skins or oily T-panels. It is generally applied before foundation, and immediately creates a matte effect. The skin is also kept matte for far longer periods than can be achieved by using powder. You may not readily find this product at your local beauty counter, but it can usually be obtained from a professional make-up supplier (see page 95).

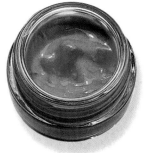

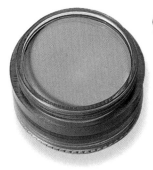

green colour corrector

The most commonly used colour corrector is green. It functions in a similar way to concealer, but the green colour is far more effective in counteracting redness in the skin, as in the case of blemishes, broken veins, or very ruddy cheeks, for example. Your usual concealer is then applied over the colour corrector.

liquid eyeliner

This product can be used instead of pencil eyeliner, but on the top lid only. A liquid eyeliner creates a much stronger, more definite line, but should preferably be kept for dramatic evening applications and then used only if you can achieve a very straight, clean line (see page 70).

eyelash thickener

This almost transparent coating is used to thicken and lengthen the eyelashes before mascara is applied.

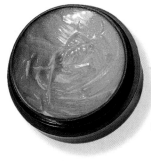

lip gloss

To add extra shine to your lips, use lip gloss. It is available in tinted or colourless formulations and can be used alone or over lipstick. It is not recommended for use on mature skin, as it tends to 'bleed' into any little lines around the lips.

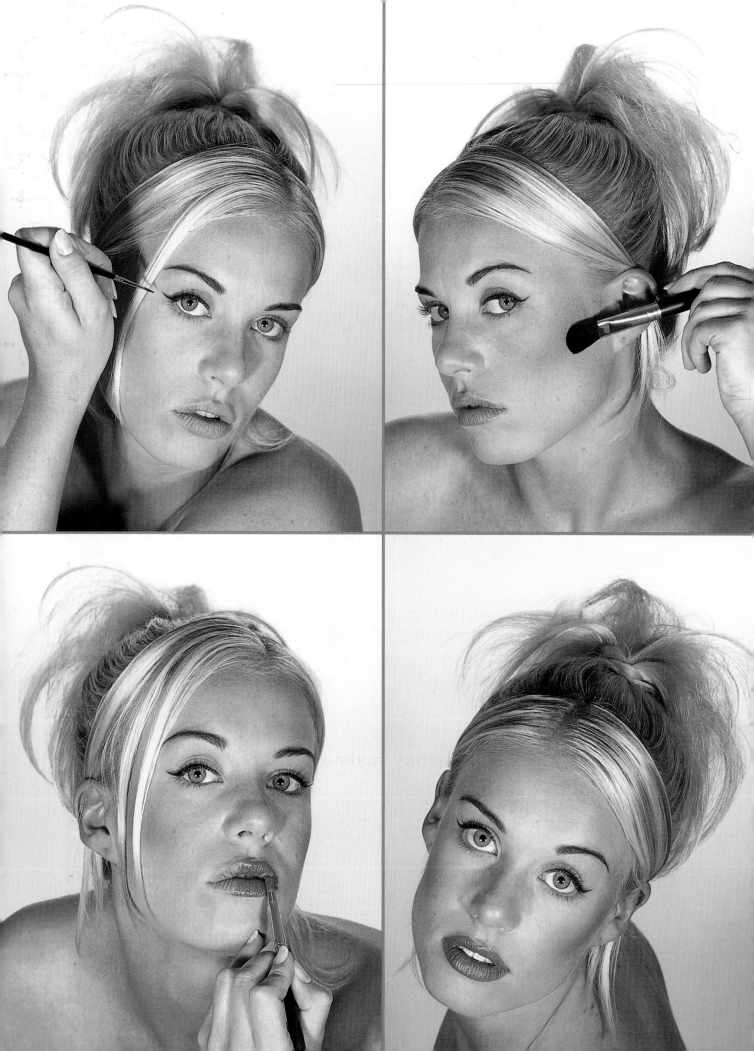

techniques

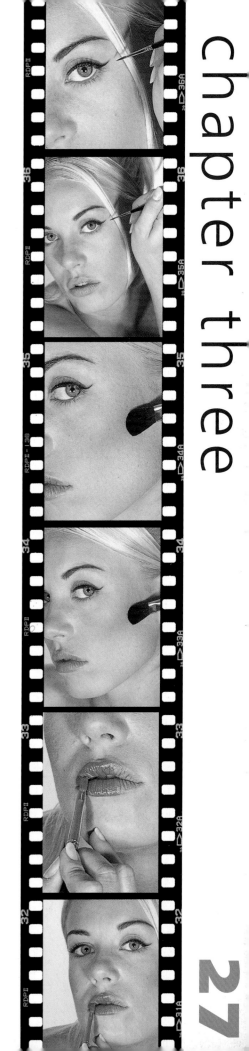

Once you have discovered which

make-up tools to use, and understand how

each make-up product functions, you can

move on to mastering various make-up

techniques. By combining the correct

tools, products and techniques you can

create any look you desire.

eyebrows
shape up

Make-up artists regard eyebrows as the most important feature of a woman's face. If your eyebrows are shapeless and untidy, they can ruin any make-up effect you try to create. If you have been neglecting your eyebrows – not realizing their significance – study this section carefully, paying particular attention to the instant 'eye-lift' illusion which is illustrated below.

The aim of removing hair from the eyebrow area is not only to thin out and neaten brows, but also to create a shape that enhances the eye. Many women pluck their eyebrows, but do not achieve a shape allowing them to create balance and illusion around the eye. Make sure that you have a clear idea of the shape you wish to achieve by studying all the photographs and illustrations in this section. Only then pick up a pair of tweezers.

the 'eye-lift' illusion

In the photograph below the eyebrow on the right has been carefully plucked to create a beautiful, arched shape. The eyebrow on the left has been left in its natural state. Look at the illusion of 'lift' created on the side of the face where the eyebrow has been shaped. The area above the eye has been opened up, providing a clear space above the lid to be shadowed cleverly, and a face that will look much more elegantly finished.

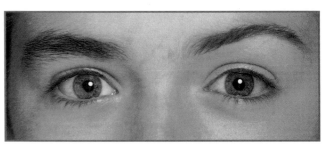

If you want to make the most of your looks, do not neglect your eyebrows. Look at the illusion of 'lift' created by removing hair from the eyebrow on the right.

the ideal eyebrow shape

As a guide to achieving the ideal eyebrow shape, look at the photograph below, and imagine similar lines being drawn across your own face.

A The thickest part – where the eyebrow begins – should be close to a point on a vertical line running roughly from the outside of the nose up towards the forehead.

B The outside of the eyebrow should end at a point on a line running from the corner of the nose past the outer corner of the eye.

C If you divide the length of the eyebrow into three equal sections, the highest point of the arched shape should be approximately two thirds outwards from the starting point.

Note that the eyebrow shape stretches up and outwards in a straight line and thins out on its decline. Any hair growing outside this desired shape is removed. It is a good idea to use a dark eyebrow pencil to practise drawing this shape over or through your brows as they currently are. If you find yourself having drawn an unsatisfactory shape, clean off the pencilled markings and start afresh. Make sure that you have achieved two more or less equal, balanced brow shapes (i.e. so that your two eyebrows match each other as closely as possible in shape) before you begin removing any hair.

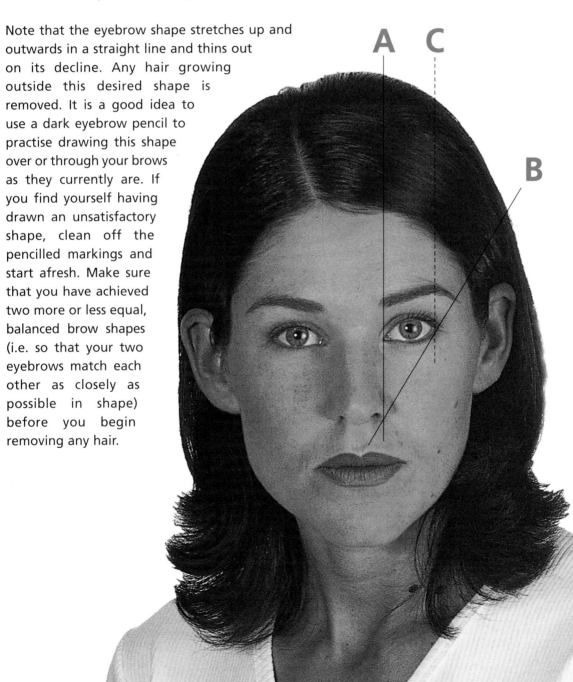

where to begin

Some women have been taught that only the outsides of the eyebrows (i.e. the area furthest from the nose) should be plucked to create an arch. They have been told that the start of the eyebrow (i.e. closest to the nose) should never be touched. Used on thick, heavy eyebrows, however, this practice will result in an unbalanced eyebrow shape. The start of the eyebrow will seem too heavy, and the shape will not create the desired illusion of 'lift' around the eye. This is a common mistake made when plucking to remove hair, so examine the diagrams below carefully.

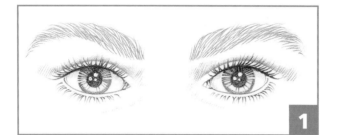

1 Here are the eyebrows in their natural state, before any hair has been removed.

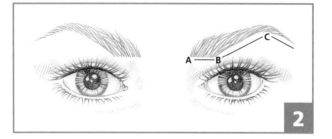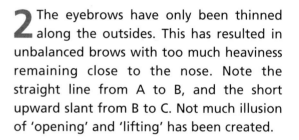

2 The eyebrows have only been thinned along the outsides. This has resulted in unbalanced brows with too much heaviness remaining close to the nose. Note the straight line from A to B, and the short upward slant from B to C. Not much illusion of 'opening' and 'lifting' has been created.

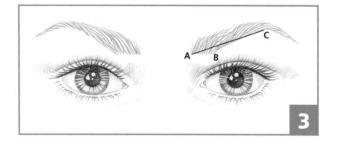

3 By connecting points A and C with a straight line and removing the hair below the line at corner B, a significant improvement can be achieved. Note how a much longer upward slant is achieved with the creation of one unbroken line stretching from A to C.

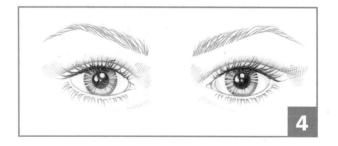

4 This is the final shape to be aimed for. Significantly more space has been opened up between the eye and the eyebrow, creating the desired illusion of 'lift'. The shape of the eyebrow now consists of one long, unbroken line stretching up to the peak, and then gently sloping down.

thinly plucked eyebrows

If you are already in the habit of plucking your eyebrows quite thinly, or if your eyebrows are naturally thin, you may still be able to improve on their shape by plucking.

1 The first photograph shows eyebrows that have already been plucked thinly. A better shape can still achieved, however, by further shaping at the start of the eyebrow (as indicated in the illustrations opposite).

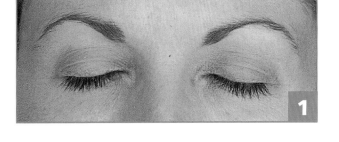

2 This photograph shows just a small amount of hair having been removed. The eyebrow shape is more balanced and the effect is far more professional.

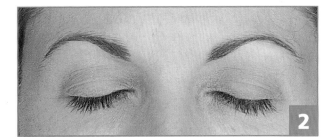

3 The final photograph shows the elegant new shape created once the eyebrows are defined with a little dark brown shadow.

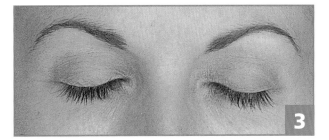

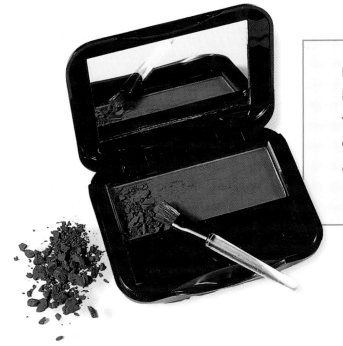

Do not judge the look of your brows when you have just plucked them, and not yet defined them. Once you have defined them with dark shadow, you will have a far better idea of the finished effect.

how to pluck

Always bear in mind that no-one has two perfectly symmetrical eyebrows. You will have to work with the natural hair growth of each brow in turn, achieving as symmetrical and even a look as possible. Defining brows with shadow or pencil after plucking can create the illusion of symmetry.

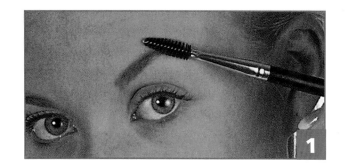

1 Using an eyebrow brush or a mascara wand, brush all the eyebrow hair on both eyebrows diagonally upwards.

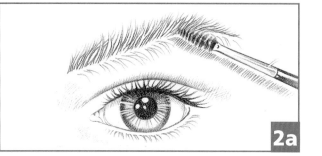

2a Now you can 'part' the brow hair as shown, brushing the hair to be removed downwards. The hair brushed upwards will not be plucked, and will form the final desired shape.

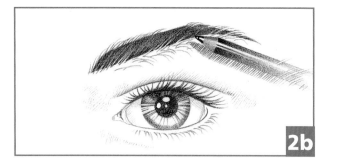

2b Alternatively, you can use a dark eyebrow pencil, or even a black eye-liner pencil, to draw in the desired eyebrow shape through the existing hair. Exaggerate the shading considerably, so that the desired shape is clearly visible. Any hair outside the shaded area will then be removed.

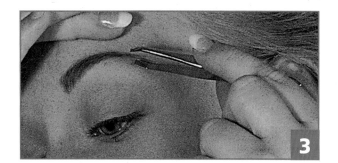

3 You now need to remove the unwanted hair. Hold the tweezers in one hand, and use the other hand to lightly stretch the skin of the area you are about to tweeze. Grasp each hair as close to its root as possible, and pluck in the direction of the natural hair growth. Work carefully, ensuring that you do not remove hair unnecessarily.

uneven eyebrows

It is normal to have uneven hair growth along the length of the eyebrow. There may be patches where hair growth is sparse, and patches where the hair is thicker. You may also, for instance, have thick, full brows at the start, and almost no hair where the brow ends towards the temples.

When it comes to applying your make-up, either an eyebrow pencil or shadow may be used to even out the appearance of brows. This technique is explained and illustrated on pages 44–47.

1 These uneven eyebrows have not yet been shaped.

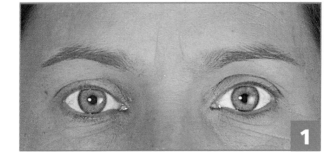

2 Now unwanted hair has been removed and the desired shape has been created.

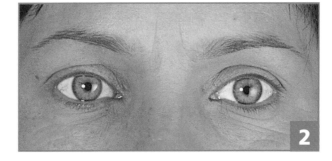

3 The final result is achieved by subtly shading the brows to provide definition and a neat, elegant finish. Note how any uneven patches have been filled in.

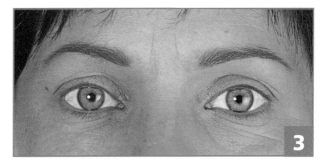

If you prefer visiting a beauty salon, make sure that the beauty therapist has a clear idea of what you want. You may wish to pencil in the desired eyebrow shape yourself, and ask for only the hair outside this shape to be removed, or take this book along as a guide to explaining the shape.

foundation, concealer & powder
create the base

Every woman I know would love to have perfect skin, but for the vast majority of us this is an impossible dream. Even the most beautiful models that appear in glossy magazines have 'imperfections' that require concealing, or have their photographs retouched before publication.

By learning the art of correctly applying foundation, concealer and powder, however, many women will find it possible to create the *illusion* of a near perfect skin tone. When I discuss the 'art' of applying these three basic products, I am referring to the technique of applying them *without making it obvious to others* that you have applied anything. The effect to strive for is to even out your skin tone – covering or minimizing imperfections – and to create a silky smooth texture on the skin. The most important factor when choosing foundation, concealer and powder is that, once applied, the products look 'invisible' and natural, like 'true skin'. To achieve this effect, it is essential to find the *exact* colours to match your individual skin tone (see page 22 for a discussion of yellow correctors). Some women dislike any form of foundation, either because they experience a 'caked' feel on the skin, or because they fear that wearing foundation will cause blocked pores. Nowadays, however, there are such advanced formulations that you will hardly be aware that you have applied anything to your skin. Carefully select foundation suited to your skin type, and you are sure to be pleased with the result. Many foundation products actually protect the skin from pollutants in the air, and contain sunscreen as well.

Some women apply foundation, but do not use powder to create a silky finish. Many women regard concealer as a product meant only for covering teenage spots or severe blemishes. In order to achieve a truly professional make-up finish, though, *all three* products are necessary. It is essential to realize that make-up will not last on the skin unless it has a properly prepared surface to cling to. Blushers and eye shadows are not formulated to work directly on the skin, or to be applied directly over foundation.

This section explains how to create a base for the application of additional make-up products. Note that your choice of product formulations will determine the order of application, as liquid or creamy products are generally followed by drier ones.

foundation

There are two very important aspects to consider when selecting foundation, namely the texture and the colour.

texture

The properties and functions of various foundation formulations (liquids, creams and powders) were discussed on pages 18–19. Experiment with textures from different make-up houses, until you find one you like. Some women like a light, 'barely there' feel on the skin, while others prefer heavier coverage. For some women the most important criteria are that a foundation is quick and easy to apply.

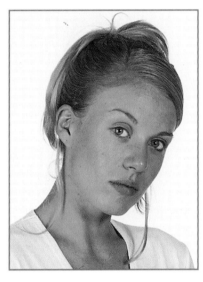

Without foundation unevenness in skin tone and patchiness are visible.

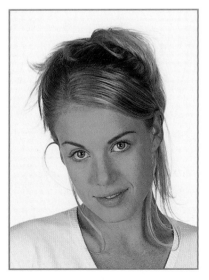

Foundation, concealer and powder create an even skin tone.

colour

This is the single most important factor in choosing foundation. If you fail to find an exact colour match for the base you are creating, you cannot expect any of the additional make-up products to contribute to enhancing the look in the way they should.

Do not leave the colour selection up to the saleslady behind the counter. Be assertive, and insist on checking the colour match carefully yourself. Salesladies are rarely professionally trained make-up artists and are generally geared to selling a particular brand of make-up. Although they may well help you find the closest foundation colour to your skin tone, this is not good enough. What you require is an *exact match*.

The lighting used in department stores also alters colours slightly. A colour that may seem like an exact match inside the store, may be far from ideal once it is seen in natural light. Always, therefore, try to find some natural light in which to check the colour before embarking on an expensive purchase.

Finally, most women go shopping when they have already applied foundation to their skins. In this case, even the most well-intentioned saleslady will find it difficult to identify the true skin tone underneath the foundation. So be brave when going shopping for foundation, and bare your natural skin tone.

The photograph on the left illustrates the application of foundation, concealer and powder matched to the skin tone exactly. Light cover has been applied just to even out the skin tone, and the look is still completely fresh and natural.

testing foundation colour

You may have to test various foundation colours before you find an exact match to your skin. Persevere, however, as a hasty or wrong choice can spoil a look completely. Take a small mirror with you for checking the colour in natural light. Once you have found the correct colour, make a note of the name so that future buys will be simple.

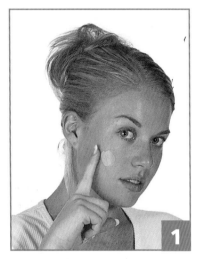

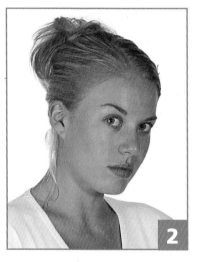

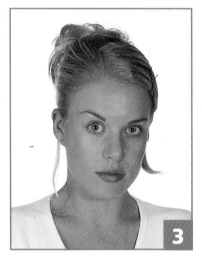

1 Begin your test with a clean skin without any make-up whatsoever, and preferably wait at least 10 minutes after having applied moisturizer. Then dot a small amount of foundation on your fingertip and apply it to your lower cheek area as shown above.

2 Now blend the foundation completely on the cheek. Move to a spot near a window or another source of natural light, and scrutinize the colour of the foundation on your skin in your mirror. Check that the light is evenly distributed across both sides of the face. The correct colour foundation should look next to 'invisible' once applied to the skin.

3 The photograph above shows the right side of the face left bare of foundation, and foundation in the correct colour applied to the left side. Notice how the foundation has not changed the natural skin colour in any way. It has evened out the skin tone quite dramatically, though.

If the colour of the foundation is at all visible, it is incorrect and you will have to start afresh. The photograph on the right demonstrates the wrong colour being used and, although this example has been exaggerated to make a point, you will be amazed at how many women are this careless when selecting foundation.

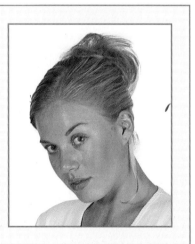

mixing foundation colours

If, when testing, you find a texture that you like, but one colour in the range is too light and the next too dark, consider your own personal mix. Provided you keep to products from the same make-up house, this may very well do the trick. I find that I inevitably have to buy two different

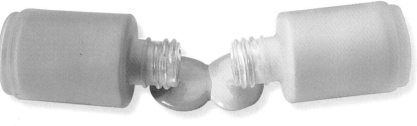

shades, take them home and mix them into a third bottle to obtain my exact colour match. I only mix a certain amount from each bottle into the third, because my skin tends to be paler in winter than in summer, when I spend a little time in the sun.

achieving a balance between pink and yellow

A common problem when testing foundation is that a colour may not seem either too pale or too dark, but still does not provide an exact match. In most cases the reason is that the foundation colour is too pink to look like true skin. In fact, the majority of us have skin with yellowy tones, and many commercial foundations simply do not contain enough yellow colouring. You will therefore see many women wearing a pinkish foundation, whilst the skin on their neck and shoulders is clearly yellow-toned. Try to avoid this at all costs, as in these cases foundation looks really artificial.

In the photograph below right, a yellow colour corrector (see page 22) has been added to the foundation to achieve an exact match to the skin tone. Do not be afraid to add yellow, as applying a little too much yellow is still better than walking around with a noticeably pink tint to the face.

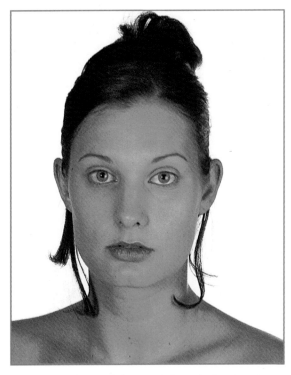

Incorrect – here pink-toned foundation has been applied to yellow-toned skin.

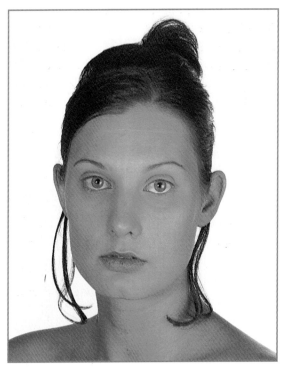

Correct – here yellow-toned foundation has been carefully matched to yellow-toned skin.

applying liquid foundation

It is best to get into the habit of applying moisturizer about 10 minutes before beginning your make-up application. If your skin still feels dry before you start applying foundation, apply a tiny amount of moisturizer to the dry areas. Then use a tissue to blot any excess before proceeding.

As liquid foundation and liquid concealer are both moist products, the order in which they are applied can vary. I prefer applying foundation first, and then only concealing what the foundation has not already covered. In addition, if concealer is applied first, there is always a chance that some of it will be wiped off as the foundation is blended across the skin.

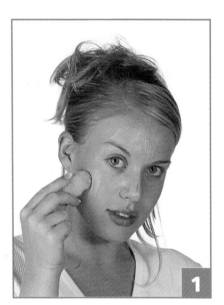

1 Foundation may be applied using a finger, but for a more even application and a natural finish I recommend using a small, natural sea sponge (see page 9). Wet the sponge first, squeeze out the excess water and then use the damp sponge to spread the foundation evenly across your face. Do not 'dab' foundation on in patches before spreading it, as some foundations dry very quickly, creating an uneven texture.

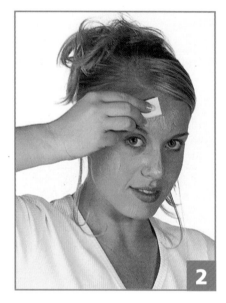

2 After spreading the foundation, use a dry or slightly damp wedge-shaped latex sponge (see page 9) to blend away any fine streaks. Also make sure that the foundation is blended into the indentations around the nose and the eye sockets, and blend carefully just around the edge of the jaw. Eyelids should be covered by foundation, but taking the foundation onto the lips is optional.

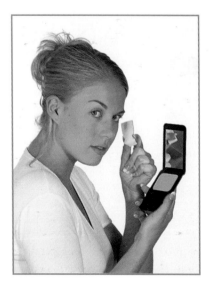

applying powder foundation

If you are using a powder-based foundation formula, you are in fact combining foundation and powder in one product. You will therefore only require concealer in addition to this, and will not need to follow the powdering process outlined on page 43.

Remember that although there are no hard-and-fast rules when it comes to applying make-up, the general rule for the order in which products are used during an application, is to apply moist products first, followed by the drier or powdery products. If you are working with a powder foundation, therefore, you will be applying concealer first (see pages 40–42).

Then, using a latex sponge, gently spread the dry foundation across the entire face. Include the eyelids, exclude the lips and blend the edges just below the jaw.

applying cream foundation

When using a cream-based foundation, concealer may be applied either before or after the foundation. Once again, use a wedge-shaped latex sponge and light strokes to apply the foundation across the face.

Be careful – many women achieve good coverage by using a cream-based foundation, but seldom achieve a finish which looks like true skin. You may feel that you have covered all your flaws and enhanced your look, whereas you may only have created a noticeably heavy and artifical 'mask' which draws attention. Had you not tried to cover everything, and applied lighter coverage, you may have found a much more pleasing natural look. You will be surprised how few people notice the flaws you worry about. Let me repeat that if people notice your make-up before anything else, you have defeated the purpose of wearing it.

for dark skin tones

For dark skins, the principles for testing colour and texture, and for applying foundation remain the same. The colours used will obviously be much darker. If parts of your face are more darkly pigmented than others, you may need to use more than one foundation colour, blending to an even look.

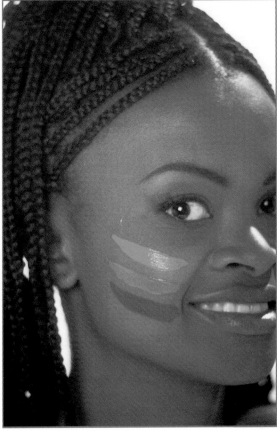

A perfect match on dark skin is very important, as anything even slightly lighter will 'grey' the skin.

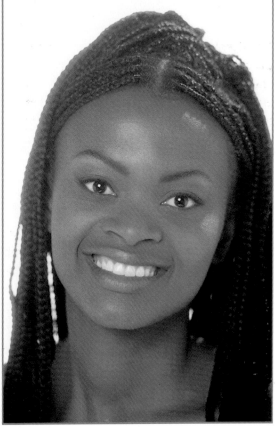

The correct foundation colour evens out the skin tone, whilst retaining a completely natural look.

concealer

Concealer is used on the areas of the face that require more cover than that provided by foundation alone. Applied to eyelids, it also offers a wonderful base for eye shadow, helping it last throughout the day.

choosing concealer

Concealers are available in a various formulations (see page 20). The kind of concealer you choose will depend on what you wish to conceal. For blemishes, a dry stick concealer may be useful, but around the eye area you need a softer product which can be applied without tugging at the skin. Professional make-up artists generally prefer using tubs of cream concealer, which are highly versatile. If you are unable to find this product in a store near you, you may wish to contact a professional supplier (see page 95) to obtain some.

where to apply concealer

A Cover the entire area from the eyelid to the eyebrow

B Mask dark rings under the eyes, staying close to the nose

C Cover any redness still visible through the foundation

D Cover any blemishes

E Avoid applying concealer to this area, as fine lines or wrinkles become emphasized

dark rings & eyelids

Every face – even a young one – is given a fresher appearance by applying concealer to the darker skin or 'ring' under the eye, as well as to the eyelids. The skin tone here often seems darker or uneven, owing either to pigmentation or because of the blood in the tiny vessels beneath the skin showing through. To apply concealer, use a soft brush (see page 13) or your finger, if you prefer.

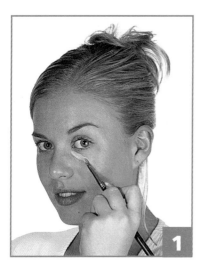

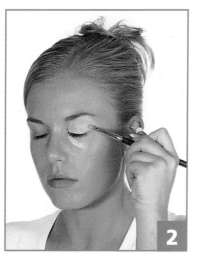

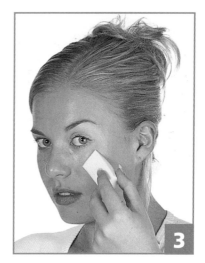

1 Using a small brush, apply concealer below the eyes close to the nose, avoiding the lined area further outwards. The darkest part of the 'ring' is usually at this inner point.

2 Then apply concealer to the entire eyelid as shown above. Extend it all the way up to the eyebrow.

3 To create a neat finish, use a wedge-shaped latex sponge to blend gently.

blemishes

To conceal a blemish or anything prominent, like a mole, for instance, apply concealer to that specific area only by using a small brush.

1 Apply only a tiny dot of concealer, using a small, firm brush made of sable hair.

2 Pat with a fingertip to blend, as a wiping motion is likely to expose whatever you have tried to cover.

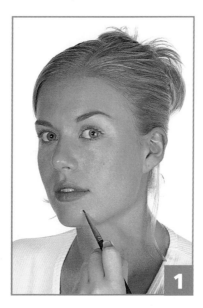

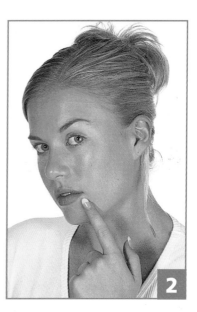

redness

If you are trying to cover a reasonably large patch of skin using concealer, it is of the utmost importance to follow the steps I have outlined below.

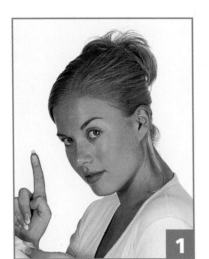

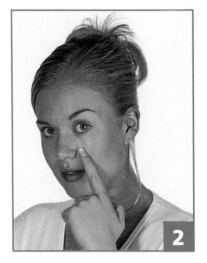

1 Use a light pat to pick up some concealer on your fingertip. Then pat your finger against a tissue to retain only a tiny amount of concealer.

2 Now very gently pat the concealer onto the reddish area, using a motion similar to combining a pat and a wipe.

As so little concealer is applied at a time, no blending should be required. If you have covered an area too heavily, however, use a wedge-shaped sponge to blend lightly.

using concealer on mature skin

Work very carefully when applying concealer to mature skin. A heavy application will not hide lines, but emphasize them instead. Ensure that you choose a soft concealer that blends easily without tugging at the skin. I recommend cream concealers (see page 20).

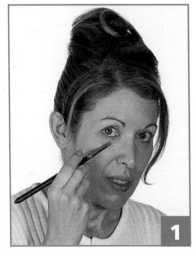

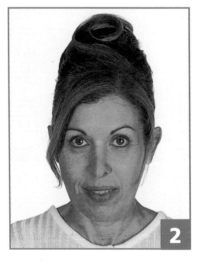

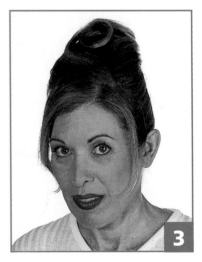

1 Use a small brush, and apply a little concealer below the eyes close to the nose, just avoiding the lined area further outwards.

2 Also apply concealer to the entire eyelid to act as a base for eye shadow. Use a latex wedge to blend gently, creating an even look.

3 The illusion of an even skin tone has been created and a fresher, more youthful look has been achieved.

powder

Applying foundation and concealer can leave the face shiny and a little sticky. The shine can make one look tired, and a sticky surface is not what you need as a base for eye shadow and blusher. Unless you have used a powder-based foundation (see page 19), applying powder is the logical next step. Powder 'sets' the foundation and gives the face a fresh, matte appearance. Not only does it act as a silky base for the application of other products, but it also helps them last. Pressed powder is less messy to carry in your handbag, but does tend to 'build up' on the skin, unlike loose powder. Used with care, it can be useful for quick touch-ups.

testing powder colour

Although powders are often labelled 'translucent', this does not mean that they are colourless. Aways test powder on your face and check that is does not alter the colour of your foundation. It is a good idea to apply foundation over the entire face, powder only half the face, and then compare the colour. Truly translucent powders are best ordered from professional suppliers (see page 95). Some companies now manufacture a yellow powder (see page 22) that is suitable for use on almost any skin tone, with the exception of very fair skin. This move towards using yellow-toned products is the best way of obtaining a next-to-natural finish.

applying loose powder

Apply a minimal amount of powder to lined areas, and remember to apply powder to the eyelids to create a smooth, silky surface for eye shadow.

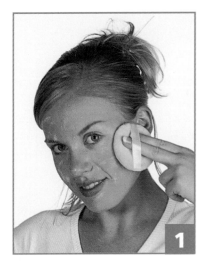 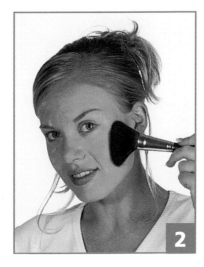 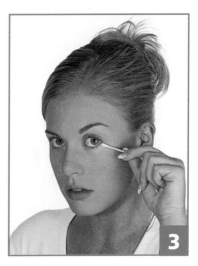

1 Using a good powder puff, apply loose powder in a gentle pressing action to set the foundation.

2 Then use a large, soft powder brush to dust off any excess powder.

3 Using a cotton bud, apply a small amount of powder under the bottom eyelashes. Your eyeliner will blend more easily and last longer.

eyebrows
gain definition

As already discussed on pages 28–33, make-up artists regard eyebrows as a very important facial feature. I discussed and illustrated how to shape eyebrows effectively by removing unwanted hair to create a flattering arch. Refresh your memory, if you like, by referring to this earlier section again, paying special attention to what I termed the 'eye-lift' illusion (see page 28).

In this section I shall be discussing and illustrating make-up application techniques to add definition to eyebrows that have already been shaped correctly by plucking. After applying foundation, concealer and powder to the face (see pages 34–43), the next step is to define the eyebrows.

The order in which the various steps of the make-up application process are followed, is very important. Experiment with a different order if you like, but I think you will find that defining your eyebrows before you proceed to the eyes, cheeks and lips makes a substantial difference in determining the overall 'balance' you aim to create.

Trends in terms of desired eyebrow colour – and even shape – may vary from time to time. There was a time when it was highly fashionable to pluck eyebrows to a very thin line. Some make-up artists working on blonde models bleach the eyebrow hair to achieve very pale, almost invisible brows. In this section I have not attempted to follow specific trends, but rather to set out techniques that are timeless and elegant, and that will suit every woman's face.

If you are not used to applying make-up of any kind to your eyebrows, you may initially feel that your make-up has been 'overdone' or that your eyebrows have been exaggerated too much by the shadow or pencil used to add definition. Always remember, however, that you will be used to seeing your 'old' look when looking in the mirror, and that you are seldom immediately able to objectively judge a 'new' look. Study the faces and the techniques used in this section carefully, and then decide whether you agree that defining eyebrows is important.

Some women may indeed be lucky enough to have thick, full, even eyebrows that require no further defining by make-up. Most of us, however, either have eyebrows that require defining throughout because of sparse, fine hair, or have sparse patches along the length of the brow that require filling in to create an even look.

the importance of defining the eyebrows

Let us begin by seeing what a face looks like without any eyebrows at all (see below left). Do you agree that it looks unbalanced? In the photograph in the centre below, the eyebrows have been included. The eyebrow on the right has been defined, while the eyebrow on the left has been left undefined. Decide for yourself which half of the face looks more balanced and finished.

Even when you opt for a more natural look, with a paler lipstick colour (see below right), the eyebrows still require defining. Again compare the separate halves of the face.

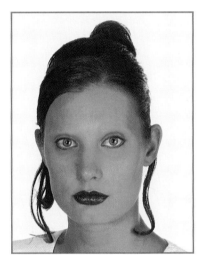

A face without eyebrows looks unbalanced – do you agree?

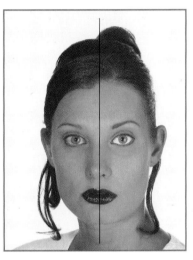

One eyebrow has been defined. Compare the overall balance.

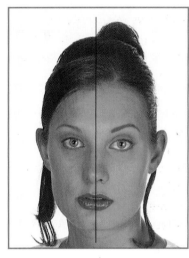

Definition is important, even when creating a more natural look.

choosing colour for your eyebrows

Your present hair colour, whether it be natural, highlighted, coloured, or sun-bleached, will determine the colour you choose for eyebrow make-up.

 Most make-up artists tend to work with black for those with black or dark brown hair.

 Dark brown is used on those with medium to dark brown hair, red hair, or mousy brown to blonde hair.

Ash-brown is used on those with blonde or very fair hair.

 Rust-brown is only used if the hair is orange-red.

 Charcoal or grey is only used on those with grey hair.

using shadow to define the brows

Unless your eyebrows are very sparse, experiment with using matte, dark eye shadow to define them. In the case of very sparse eyebrows, I recommend using eyebrow pencils (see page 22). In terms of texture, choose eye shadow that does not easily break into dust, or you may risk a rather messy application.

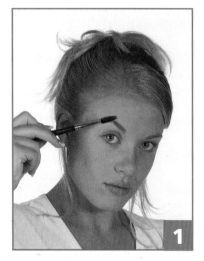 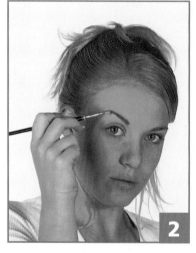 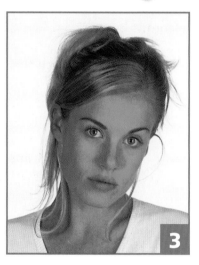

1 First brush the eyebrows into place using a special eyebrow brush or a clean wand-type applicator.

2 Use a small brush of sable hair, or a narrow, angled brush to ensure a neat finish. Lightly dip the brush into the eye shadow. Apply very little powder at a time, dusting off most of the powder you pick up onto a tissue. The real art of defining eyebrows lies in the application of multiple, light, sweeping strokes, thus gradually building up colour to create a natural finish.

3 Working with your natural eyebrow shape and hair growth, aim to achieve a shape which is as close as possible to the ideal. Notice how all the 'gaps' have been filled in and the eyebrow has an even colour throughout.

If your eyebrow hair refuses to retain the shape into which you comb it, use a tiny amount of hairspray on your eyebrow brush.

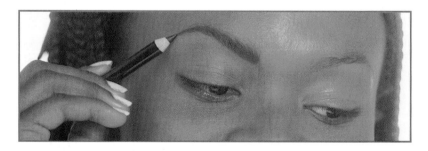

for dark skin tones

Darker skins need a stronger eyebrow than one created by using eye shadow. I recommend using a sharp, hard, dry eyebrow pencil in black. Compare the full-face photograph on page 39 (right).

using eyebrow pencil to define the brows

If you have very little eyebrow hair, applying eye shadow as described on the previous page will look smudgy and unnatural. Rather opt for a good eyebrow pencil (see page 22). If you do not use the correct pencilling technique, though, you may still run the risk of creating an artificial, 'painted' look.

You will be able to create truly natural-looking pencilled eyebrows by:

♦ using proper eyebrow pencils instead of pencil eyeliner
♦ using eyebrow pencils that are hard enough
♦ not applying too much pressure when pencilling
♦ not drawing one solid line.

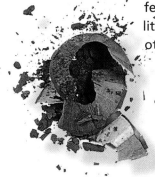

The correct way to pencil eyebrows is to use a sharp, hard, dry eyebrow pencil and apply the colour in short, light, feathery strokes, forming lots of little hair-like lines on top of each other in the desired eyebrow shape. This does require a certain degree of practice, but once you have mastered the technique, nobody will notice that your brows are not 'real'.

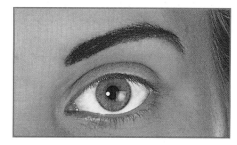

This eyebrow is far too heavily pencilled and looks obviously 'artificial'.

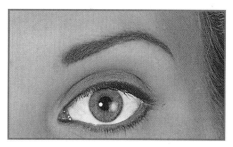

Pencilled correctly, this eyebrow looks elegant yet natural.

using two pencils

To achieve a natural look, you may want to try the technique of combining two pencils of different colours.

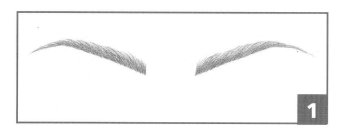

1 First pencil in a series of light, feathery strokes using a brow pencil in a colour matching that of your natural hair.

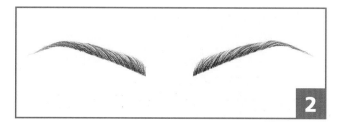

2 Then use a pencil in a slightly darker shade to distribute tiny, darker strokes throughout the length of the eyebrow as illustrated on the left. Concentrate on beginning the strokes along the baseline of the eyebrow throughout the process.

colour
on the face

Whatever your particular colouring in terms of skin tone, eyes, eyebrows and hair, there will always be certain colours that enhance your natural beauty and certain colours that detract from it. Your choice of foundation, concealer and powder, and the importance of matching it to your skin tone has already been discussed on pages 34–43. In this section I shall be discussing and illustrating the use of colour on the face in the form of make-up products like lipsticks, blushers, eyeliners and eye shadows.

For a make-up artist, adding colour to a woman's face is a tricky subject – not because it is difficult to find suitable colour combinations, but because most women grow used to applying certain colours and resist any change that may be suggested. In my experience women invariably dislike colours that they are not accustomed to seeing on their faces.

At this point I would strongly like to encourage you to experiment with different colours on your face. Unless you try out new colours from time to time, you may well become one of the many women who become slaves to the same one or two colours which they use year after year. Not only will your daily make-up application become boring, but you will miss out on the rewards of experimenting with new products and colours which appear on the shelves each season. Although new colour combinations may feel awkward at first, give yourself a chance to get used to them. You may also find that friends begin complimenting you on your looks, not realizing what you have done differently, but simply noticing that you look really good, or fresh and elegant.

'cool' and 'warm' colours

An effective way of determining which make-up colours suit you best, is to separate what we call 'cool' colour palettes from 'warm' colour palettes. Most people will find that one of these colour palettes suits them better than the other – they will either look good in 'cool' tones, or in 'warm' tones. Sometimes the difference can also be very subtle.

telling the difference

Colours that are called 'cool', are given that name because when you look at them, or when you imagine yourself surrounded by them, you experience a 'cool' feeling. So-called 'warm' colours are said to impart a 'warm' feeling. To begin training yourself to be able to look at colours and determine their 'feel' – as being either 'cool' or 'warm' – try using the simple examples given below.

The ocean – a huge mass of blue – is cool, and one can 'feel' its coolness before even touching the water. Blue is thus regarded as a 'cool' colour.

Fire – with flames of orange – is warm, and one can feel the heat without having to go anywhere near the flame. Orange is therefore regarded as a 'warm' colour.

Looking at a wider range of colours, use your imagination to 'feel' either more warmth or more coolness in a colour. Mauve, for example, echoes more of the cool 'ocean' feel than the warm 'fire' feel. Mauve is also closer in colour to blue than it is to orange, and so mauve is regarded as a 'cool' colour. Moving further along the spectrum, one can look at a pink colour. We know that pink is close to mauve, therefore one can say that pink also belongs to the 'cool' group of colours. Yellow, on the other hand, evokes more of the warm 'fire' feel than the cool 'ocean' feel. It is also closer in colour to orange than it is to blue, so yellow can be classified as a 'warm' colour.

When working with make-up, it is a little more complicated to divide colours into 'cool' and 'warm' groups, because instead of looking at simple primary and secondary colours, one uses various make-up 'neutrals' to create illusions on the face. The blusher colours on this page, for example, have been specially selected – the blusher at the top being cool, and the one below being warm. We could simply have chosen pink as cool and orange as warm, but these more 'neutral' blusher colours clearly illustrate the subtle difference between 'cool neutrals' and 'warm neutrals'.

A particular skin tone will either look better combined with cool make-up colours, or with warm make-up colours. If your skin tone is best suited to cool colours, your skin will be referred to as having a blue undertone. On the other hand, if your skin tone is best suited to warm colours, your skin will be referred to as having a yellow undertone.

what suits you?

When discussing foundation, concealer and powder on pages 34–43, I spoke of most people as having a yellow surface tone to their skin, and therefore sometimes having to add yellow products to their foundation to achieve a perfect match to their particular skin tone. At this point, however, it is important to clearly distinguish between the 'surface tone' and the 'undertone' of the skin. These two terms refer to different qualities of the skin. Although it may sound contradictory, the majority of us have a yellow surface tone, but a blue undertone.

Clients who consult me professionally often inform me that they have already determined their 'colour type', having, for instance, analyzed the colour of the skin on the inside of their forearms. Quite often, however, they have made an inaccurate assessment, because they have been looking at the yellow of their skin's surface tone instead of the skin's particular undertone.

To help solve this problem, I suggest that you use pages 52 and 53 in this book, as well as two rather bright lipstick colours (see below right) to conduct a very practical test.

doing 'the colour test'

When you conduct this test, make sure that your face is evenly lit by natural light. Try standing near a window, but not in bright or direct sunlight. Use a mirror large enough for you to see your whole face, including the neck and shoulders. Bare your shoulders, as a coloured garment may influence your perception of the colours you are testing.

Your skin should be bare of all make-up, including foundation, concealer and powder. Do not cover any uneven patches, blotches or red veins – if left uncovered they will, in fact, assist you. Pin or tie your hair back to scrape it off your face completely, so that its colour does not distract you.

If you do not trust your own judgement, try doing this test in the company of a couple of good friends who will be honest and objective. Be careful when selecting someone to help you, though, as they may subconsciously choose the colour they prefer, and not the colour that suits you best.

To do the test, you will compare orange and pink. It is essential that the colours used are of a similar intensity, though, or your judgement will be inaccurate. You will need an orange and a pink lipstick similar to those shown above, as well as pages 52 and 53 of this book.

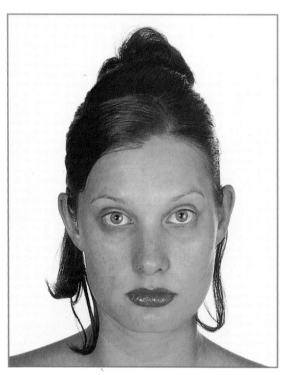

A cool undertone with the wrong *colour.*

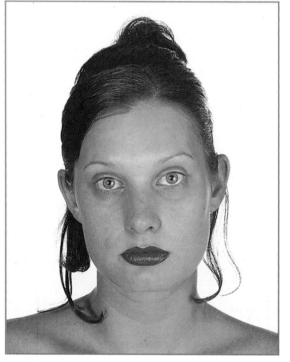

A cool undertone with the correct *colour.*

step-by-step

1 Turn the book and hold it so that the pink page (page 52) is below your chin, and the orange page (page 53) is hanging down towards the floor. Look at your face in the mirror with only the pink page next to it, paying attention to your face, not to the page of colour. See how the pink colour interacts with any imperfections like unevenness in skin tone, blotches, blemishes or red veins. Do these imperfections show up more, or do they seem to fade?

2 Now follow the same procedure again – this time holding the orange page (page 53) below your chin, with the pink page (page 52) hanging out of sight. Look at how the orange colour interacts with your skin, and with any imperfections.

3 For this step and the next, you will require lipstick. Firstly, apply the pink lipstick, and again hold the pink page next to your face. Study the effect the colour has on your appearance.

4 Use a good make-up remover to remove all traces of the pink lipstick from your lips. Then apply the orange lipstick, and hold the orange page next to your face.

The *wrong* colour will make the skin around blemishes appear paler, and make the blemishes seem more noticeable. Your skin may also look blotchy, especially around the mouth area.

The *correct* colour seems to give the skin a radiant glow and it creates a generally harmonious look, with blemishes becoming less noticeable.

The photographs on this page and the previous page illustrate the effect achieved by applying either the wrong or the correct colour to the face.

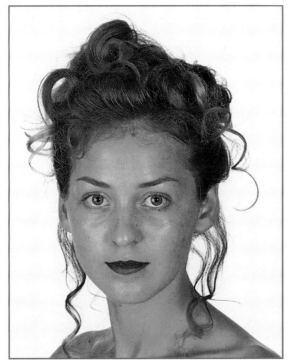

A warm undertone with the wrong colour.

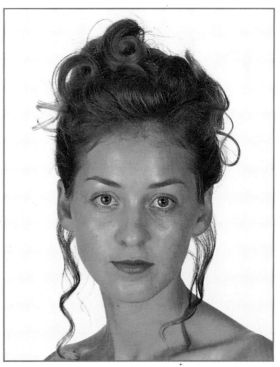

A warm undertone with the correct colour.

cool & warm 'neutrals'

It is quite easy to classify bright, clear pink and orange, like the lipsticks in tubs used on page 50, as either 'cool' or 'warm'. Page 52 of this book is also clearly 'cool', whilst page 53 is clearly 'warm'.

When it comes to making the distinction in terms of make-up colours, however, things are not that simple. To create a natural, elegant, timeless look, make-up artists do not use bright blues, greens, pinks, oranges or yellows, as these colours are too bright to create any feeling of depth on the face. To create illusion around the eyes, as well as on the cheeks and lips, make-up artists need to shade or darken certain areas to make them recede, and highlight other areas to make them seem more prominent. To do this most successfully, 'neutral' colours are used, especially on the eyes and cheeks.

Gaining an understanding of the term 'neutral' colour is therefore essential – as is being able to see the difference between a 'cool neutral' colour and a 'warm neutral' colour. Looking at a range of neutral colours, like different shades of brown, for example, and dividing them into cool and warm shades can be quite tricky. To simplify the process, I suggest asking yourself what I call 'the colour question': *Can I see more pink and mauve tones in this colour, or more orange and yellow tones?*

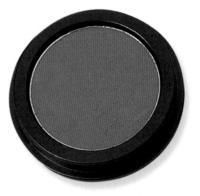

a *Pink and mauve are cool colours. This brown has subtle mauve tones, and so it belongs in a cool palette.*

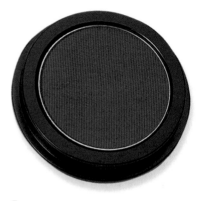

b *Orange and yellow are warm colours. This brown has subtle orange tones, and so it belongs in a warm palette.*

The same 'colour question' can be asked of these five lipstick colours.

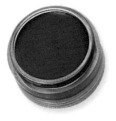 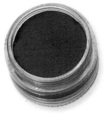 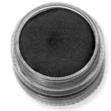 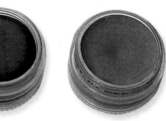

cool reds

primary red
(not influenced by
cool or warm tones
and can be worn
by everyone)

warm reds

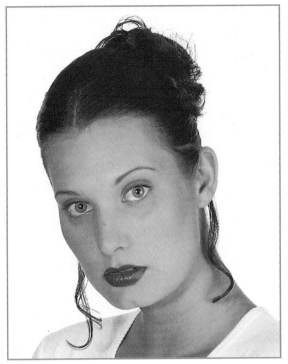

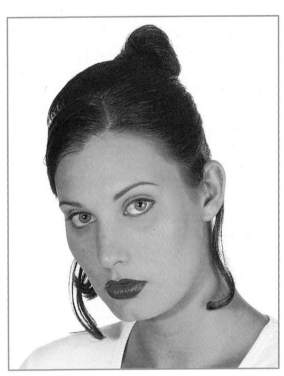

A cool undertone with the wrong colours.

A cool undertone with the correct colours.

Although certain colours may be your favourites, because you know they look good and you have become used to them, be brave enough to experiment. Once you have identified whether warm or cool colours suit you best, try some variations within the warm or cool palette. You may discover that colours you never thought of using look great on you. On the following two pages I have set out the various make-up colours I recommend in terms of warm and cool palettes.

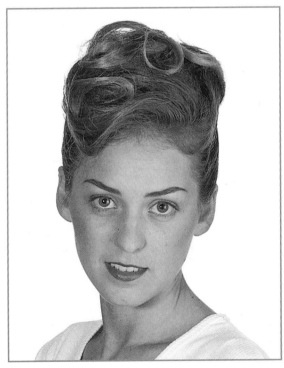

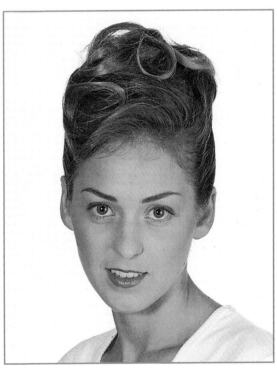

A warm undertone with the wrong colours.

A warm undertone with the correct colours.

cool

eye shadow

lipstick

blusher

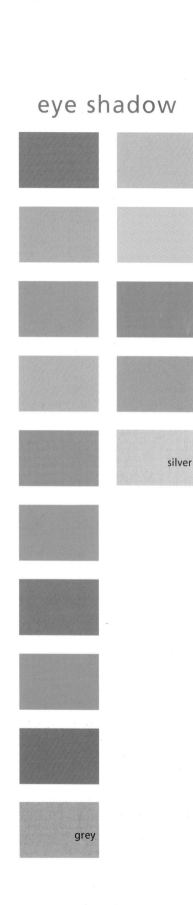

silver

grey

cool make-up colours

If you have completed 'the colour test' (see pages 50–51) and determined that your skin has a *cool* undertone, select your make-up colours from the palette set out on this page. Note that there are three categories of colours: one for eye shadows, one for lipsticks, and one for blushers. You could even consider taking these charts with you as a guide when shopping for make-up.

warm

eye shadow

lipstick

blusher

gold

warm make-up colours

If you have completed 'the colour test' (see pages 50–51) and determined that your skin has a *warm* undertone, select your make-up colours from the palette set out on this page. Note that there are three categories of colours: one for eye shadows, one for lipsticks, and one for blushers. You could even consider taking these charts with you as a guide when shopping for make-up.

eyes
do the talking

A woman's eyes are her most expressive facial feature. When we communicate, we look into each others' eyes. And eyes can be used most effectively to convey a wide range of emotions, depending on the setting – from the ballroom to the boardroom. Learning how eye make-up techniques can influence the image you project is thus very important. Keep your 'evening eyes' for glamorous occasions, and look professional, yet natural and elegant at work.

Eye make-up should be used to enhance your eyes – in terms of their colour and shape – and not to provide 'decoration'. If your eye shadow attracts more attention than your eyes themselves, the purpose of the application has been defeated. Matte, neutral shades applied in the right places will draw someone's gaze into the eyes themselves. Shimmery pale blue shadow from eyelid to eyebrow will only draw attention to itself.

Applying eye make-up is probably the trickiest of all the techniques to be mastered. Practise this part of your make-up application and learn what works for you.

the art of illusion

The key to the art of eye make-up application is being able to successfully create illusions. Any 'faults' you perceive – although other people may not regard them as such – can be minimized, and the illusion of more beautiful and youthful, bright, expressive eyes can be created. No matter whether you feel your eyes are 'too small', 'too round' or 'too deep-set' or whether you have 'too little' or 'too much' eyelid, or close-set or wide-set eyes – each of these factors will be discussed.

highlighting and shading

The two basic techniques used to enhance the eye's natural shape are *highlighting* and *shading*. Without question the most effective colours to combine with this technique are matte, neutral shades, such as those at the top of this page, namely white or cream highlighter, and a warm or cool shading colour, such as those shown above. Always bear in mind this basic rule: *light brings an area forward and makes it appear larger or more prominent, while dark makes an area recede, or makes it appear smaller and less prominent.* To create the desired illusion, it is essential to work with light and dark together.

cool   eye-shadow colours   warm

highlighters
(use any of the three pale colours
below, or any other light colours
from the cool palette)

highlighters
(use any of the three pale colours
below, or any other light colours
from the warm palette)

shading colours

shading colours

Your choice of colours for highlighting and shading is not determined by the colour of your eyes, but by determining whether your skin has a cool or warm undertone. If you have not already identified the colour of your skin undertone, do so now before continuing. The technique used to do this is set out on pages 50–51.

Blue eye shadow is most certainly not the best way of enhancing blue eyes, nor green eye shadow the best for green eyes. In fact, blue and green eye shadows are usually highly problematic, and should be used with great discretion. In this book, for instance, I have used blue only to line eyes (see page 48), and green to create a fun, funky evening look for a young girl (see page 87).

Once you have determined whether you have a cool or warm skin undertone, use the charts of cool and warm colours supplied on this page to help you select effective colours to be used for highlighting and shading. You will note that most of these colours are matte, neutral shades, but that they still offer you a wide range of choices.

Please note, also, that these are not the *only* colours I recommend – they are merely offered as a guide within the cool and warm ranges. If your favourite colour does not appear here, do not despair!

key

▼ not recommended for deep-set or small eyes
● preferably for younger skin or evening application only

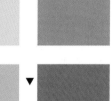

grey   silver

copper

gold

eyelid shape

Before deciding which part of the eye area to highlight and which part to shade, it is essential to examine the shape of your eyes and eyelids. Everyone can begin by applying highlighter to the browbone just below the eyebrow, but when it comes to the eyelid, one is faced with a choice. Depending on the amount of visible eyelid, you will decide whether to highlight or shade your lid. Do you want the lid to look more prominent, or less prominent? Study your eyes in a mirror and compare their shape to the illustrations below. Look straight ahead, and do not lift or drop your chin. Which illustration most closely resembles your eye, especially in terms of the shape of the lid?

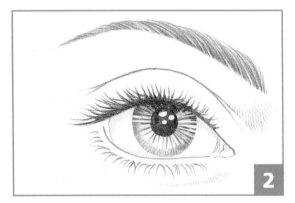

Little or no eyelid is visible.

1 If your eyes most closely resemble illustration 1 in shape, with little or no visible eyelid, you will want to create the illusion of there being more eyelid. You should therefore be applying highlighter on the lid to bring it forward and make it more prominent. You will shade only the crease of the eye, taking the shading colour outwards to join the outside corner of the eye.

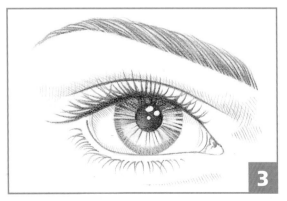

The eyelid is too prominent or puffy, or too much of it protrudes.

2 If your eyes most closely resemble illustration 2 in shape, you will want to create the illusion of there being less visible eyelid, or of it being less protruding or puffy. You should therefore be shading the lid as well as the crease of the eye. In this case, highlighter will only be applied below the eyebrow, and not on the eyelid itself.

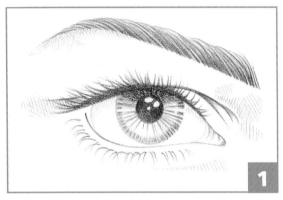

Here the ideal amount of eyelid is visible.

3 If your eyes most closely resemble illustration 3 in shape, you are lucky to have the choice of either highlighting or shading the lid area. You will still be shading the crease of the eye, and applying highlighter under the eyebrow.

using shadow to create shape

On the previous page you will have learnt how to determine whether your eyelids should be highlighted or shaded, or whether you are free to choose either highlighting or shading. I have not yet discussed the *shape* in which highlighter and shading colour should be applied, however.

To determine the shape of the shading, you need to study not the shape of the eye as before, but *the shape of the surrounding skin and bone structure.*

Study the four illustrations below, and look at the differences and the similarities between them. In illustrations a and b, the eyelids have been highlighted. In illustrations c and d, the eyelids have been shaded. Using what you have learnt about the shape of your own eyelids on the previous page, you will study either illustrations a and b, or illustrations c and d.

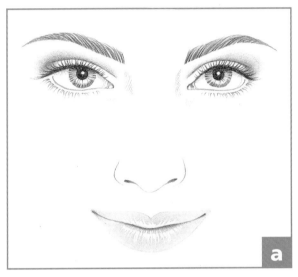

The lid is highlighted, and the crease is shaded. The shading follows the rounded crease of the lid and then comes down to the outer corner of the eye.

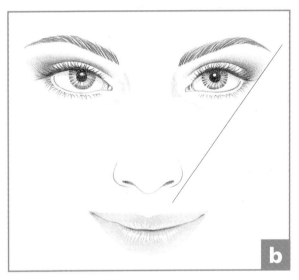

The lid is highlighted, and the crease is shaded. The shading colour extends upwards and outwards into a 'wing' shape in line with the end of the brow.

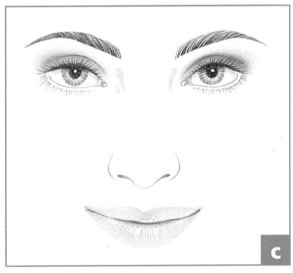

The eyelid and the crease are both shaded. The shading follows the rounded crease of the lid and then comes down to the outer corner of the eye.

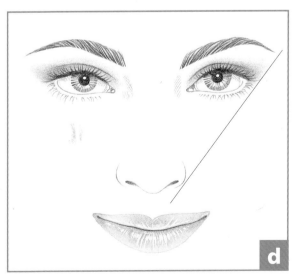

The eyelid and the crease are both shaded. The shading colour extends upwards and outwards into a 'wing' shape in line with the end of the brow.

choosing a suitable shape

The best way of finding out which of the two shapes suits you personally, is to apply the 'rounded' shading shape (either a or c on the previous page) to one eye, and the 'winged' shading shape (either b or d) to the other eye. Then compare your eyes, and decide which shape is most enhancing. You may find that you are lucky enough to be able to use either shape, and are not limited to one shape alone (i.e. you may be able to use both a and b, OR c and d, OR any of the four).

The rounded application technique (either a or c) suits most people, unless you have very little space between the crease of your eye and your eyebrow. In this case, you only have room to work outwards, so use the winged shape.

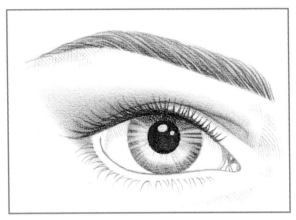

Use the winged application technique with care. It is best used on younger eyes, or where the skin towards the outside of the eye is firm and does not sag at all.

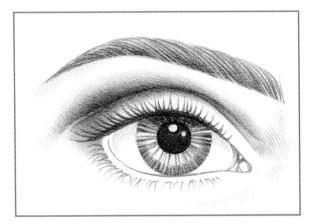

If your browbone prominently curves around the eye as illustrated above, avoid applying shadow in a winged shape.

If you have applied too much eye shadow and the colour has gone darker than you would have liked, do not rub at the colour to tone it down. Rather dip a ball of cotton wool in your loose powder and gently blend until the colour has lightened. Once you have achieved the desired shade, dust off excess loose powder.

Left: Cotton buds are very useful for neatening the edges of your eye-shadow shape, especially if you are applying shadow in the the winged shape extending outwards.

wide-set eyes and close-set eyes

If you have particularly wide-set or close-set eyes, you may want to further refine your application technique. To avoid confusion, all the illustrations below show the eyelid having been highlighted. If your eyelid is better suited to being shaded (see page 61), replace the highlighter with a shading colour. Also retain the rounded or winged shape as appropriate (see pages 61–62).

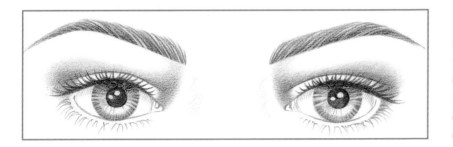

For wide-set eyes suited to the rounded application shape, extend the colour inwards from the crease and up towards the eyebrow to create the illusion of less space between the eyes.

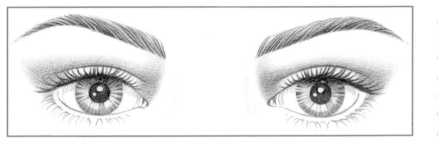

For wide-set eyes suited to the winged application shape, extend the shading colour inwards from the crease and up towards the eyebrow to create the illusion of less space between the eyes.

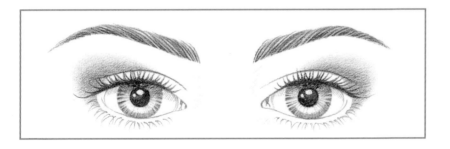

For close-set eyes suited to the rounded application shape, avoid shading the inner part of the eye crease and ensure that the shading begins and fades gently – not along hard lines.

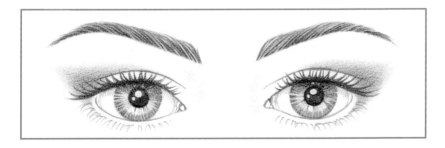

For close-set eyes suited to the winged application shape, avoid shading the inner part of the eye crease and ensure that the shading begins and fades gently – not along hard lines.

For eyes that are deep-set or small, avoid using dark shading colours (marked with a ▼ on the colour chart on page 59), as these will accentuate the 'flaws'. Keep your eyes lighter – even for evenings – and darken your blusher and lipstick.

using brushes to apply eye shadow

When using brushes to apply powder eye shadow, use a dome-shaped brush to apply the powder, and a flat-topped brush to blend hard 'edges' or 'bands' of colour. If there is not much space between the eye and the eyebrow, use a smaller brush to ease application.

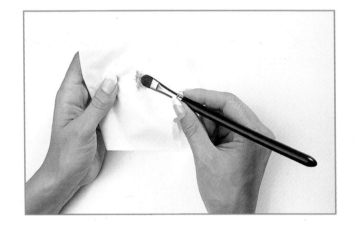

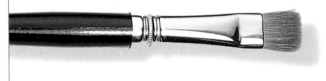

Hold the dome-shaped brush on its side as shown on the left, and gently sweep it across the shadow. This will allow the powder to be picked up evenly along the graduated shape, as it clings to the individual hairs. When the brush is swept across the skin, the powder will be spread out evenly, and not deposited only in one patch.

Always dust the excess shadow from the brush onto a tissue before bringing the brush up to your eye. If you have done this, there will be no excess powder to fall messily below the eye.

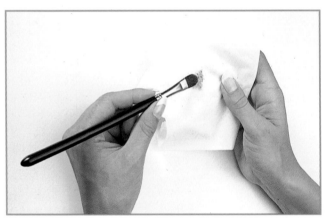

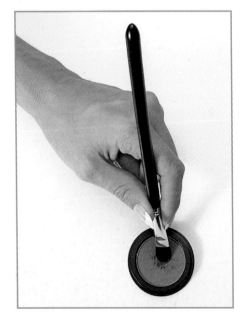

Do not 'dip' your brush into the eye shadow from the top as shown (left), as the powder will then only be picked up by the brush tip. The angle at which the brush hits the product here also causes the compacted powder to break up into small pieces. Much of the product will be wasted, and it will become increasingly difficult and messy to work with.

applying eye shadow

Remember that any eye shadow product requires a base on the skin to cling to. If you have not already done so, gently apply and blend concealer over the entire eyelid (see pages 41 and 42), and then powder well (see page 43). Make sure that the lid feels powdery and silky – not tacky – before beginning an eye-shadow application.

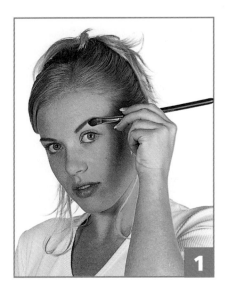

1 Using a medium to large dome-shaped brush, apply your chosen highlighter below the eyebrow.

2 Depending on the shape of your eyelid (see page 60), also apply highlighter to the lid across the bulge of the eye and all the way down to the lashes. If you will be shading your eyelid instead of high-lighting it, move on to the next stage.

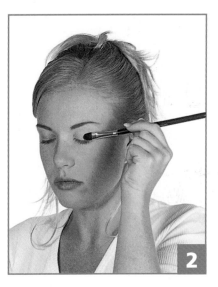

Use a smaller dome-shaped brush to apply the colour you have chosen for shading. When applying darker colours, a smaller brush is easier to work with.

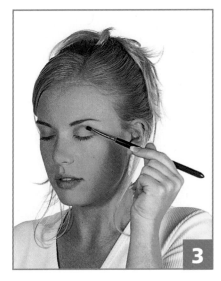

3 Using the technique described on page 61, sweep the brush along the crease of the eyelid in the curve as shown. Apply the shadow keeping the brush flat against the skin and using the entire length of the hair, not only the tip of the brush. Work the colour along the eye crease evenly. If you are shading your lid rather than highlighting it (see page 61), now also work the shadow across your eyelid all the way down to the lashes.

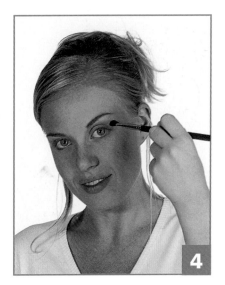

4 Now use a flat-topped brush for blending. Gently sweep across the areas where the light and dark colours meet, to blend and soften the edges as well as to even out the distribution of the eye shadow.

the importance of blending

To illustrate the importance of blending eye shadow colours after application, I have here included two photographs in which I use a combination of brown and black as shading colours.

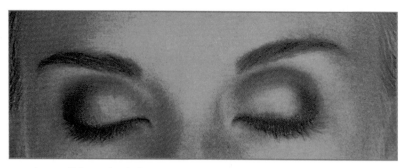

On the eyelid on the left the colours have been blended and the 'hard edges' have been softened. This is the effect to be aimed for.

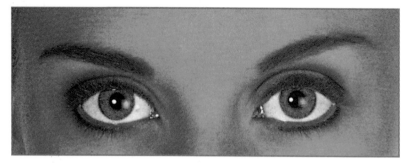

When the eyes are open, the softening effect of blending is clear. Compare the softened line below the eye on the left to the hard line on the right.

Look at the eye on the right in the top photograph. You will notice that highlighter has been applied to the brow-bone, as well as to the eyelid. The prominence of the eyelid is therefore being enhanced.

Brown eye shadow has been applied to the crease of the eye in a rounded shape, and the brown colour has been brought down in a curve to the outer corner of the eye.

Black eye shadow has been applied to the outer corner of the eyelid only, in a slightly curved shape. Note how the eye shadow does not extend beyond the outer corner. The black and brown shadows have not yet been blended on the right side, so that you are still able to distinguish the two separate colours.

using shimmer

Eye shadows containing a shimmer or pearly finish should be used with great care. For example, if a shimmer colour is applied to a puffy or wrinkled area on the eye, sparkle in the colour will illuminate the puffiness or wrinkle and make it more obvious, even though the base colour of the shimmer may be dark. Here the shimmer finish can defeat the purpose of applying dark shading, because it can draw attention to the exact area you wish to make less prominent. For mature skin, I strongly recommend keeping to matte neutrals only, to create as youthful an illusion as possible. Even on younger skins, I generally use shimmer eye shadows only for evening make-up, where lighting is less harsh than daylight, unless I am working for a magazine requiring a specific look. Using shimmer for fun, funky evening looks is discussed on pages 86–87.

using colour

As discussed and illustrated on the previous pages, I strongly recommend keeping to neutral colours like warm or cool browns to create effective illusions, yet natural-looking eye make-up. There are times, however, when some colour may be appropriate to add a little glamour. Use your discretion, though, as you do not want your eye make-up drawing more attention than your eyes.

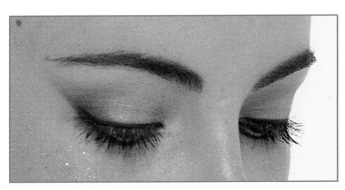

To create these funky 'evening eyes', deep purple eyeliner is used, and the colour is echoed in the extended 'wing' shape.

Evening make-up offers the best opportunity for adding colour to the eyes. In dim lighting in a restaurant or theatre, for example, the face can sometimes look rather pale and 'washed out'. Now is the time to use eye shadow in a brighter colour to frame the eyes – close to the lashes – in the same way in which you would use eyeliner. Dark blue, dark purple or dark green can be highly effective, and you will notice that I have included these colours in the colour charts for eyeliner on page 68.

'evening eyes'

The only difference between make-up techniques used to create daytime and evening looks, is that darker shading colours can be used at night. The application technique remains exactly the same. Compare the two photographs below, where a very glamorous evening look has been created using black eye shadow applied in a rounded shape.

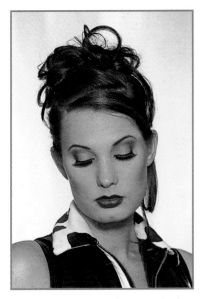

Black shadow and false eyelashes create a dramatic look.

eyeliner

The function of eyeliner is to frame and define the eyes, drawing attention to them. Note clearly that I say attention should be drawn to the eyes – not to the eye make-up. Never apply such harsh eyeliner that it draws attention to itself, rather than to the eye it is enhancing.

To line eyes subtly yet effectively, many make-up artists prefer using eye shadow instead of eye pencil. Pencils used for lining eyes should be soft and smudgy (see page 23), so that they do not drag at the delicate skin around the eye. This does mean that eyeliner pencils contain a fair amount of oil, though, which melts with heat.

A line of eye shadow is softer and easier to blend than pencil. During application there is no tugging at the skin, and shadow does not melt or smudge in humid climates as often as pencil does.

choosing eyeliner colours

Colours used to line eyes should always be subtle and, once again, the colours are determined by your natural skin tone and hair colour. In certain cases, brighter colours may be applied, but this should not become a habit, and colour should be used with great care. The chart given here indicates the range of eyeliner colours I recommend.

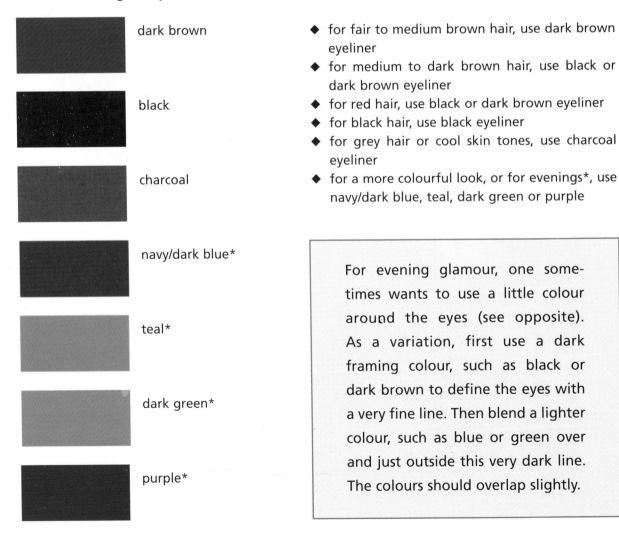

dark brown

black

charcoal

navy/dark blue*

teal*

dark green*

purple*

◆ for fair to medium brown hair, use dark brown eyeliner
◆ for medium to dark brown hair, use black or dark brown eyeliner
◆ for red hair, use black or dark brown eyeliner
◆ for black hair, use black eyeliner
◆ for grey hair or cool skin tones, use charcoal eyeliner
◆ for a more colourful look, or for evenings*, use navy/dark blue, teal, dark green or purple

For evening glamour, one sometimes wants to use a little colour around the eyes (see opposite). As a variation, first use a dark framing colour, such as black or dark brown to define the eyes with a very fine line. Then blend a lighter colour, such as blue or green over and just outside this very dark line. The colours should overlap slightly.

using eye shadow as eyeliner

When you are using eye shadow to frame the eyes, I recommend that you use a high-quality compacted powder formulation that does not break up into dust as you apply it. The dustiness is messy, and could irritate the eyes. Some make-up artists prefer working with a wet brush, but I like working with the dry shadow to ensure a soft, smoky edge and no hard lines. A small brush made of sable hair is the ideal applicator (see page 12).

applying eyeliner with a brush

The following steps will show you how and where to apply eyeliner.

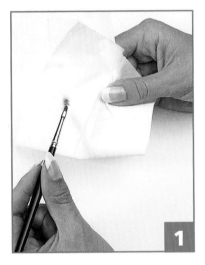 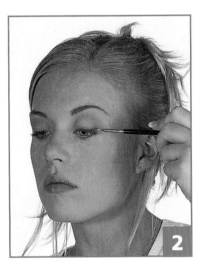 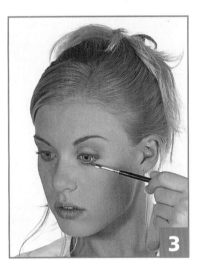

1 Always dust excess powder from the brush onto a tissue to leave very little powder on the brush.

2 Apply a line of shadow to the top lid, getting as close to the lashes as possible.

3 Apply a soft line of eye shadow under the eye, joining the top line at the outside corner.

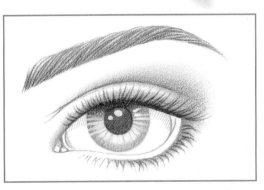

4 Use a clean cotton bud to soften any hard lines you have created.

using colour to line eyes

If you want to add some colour to your eyes on occasion, eyeliner offers the perfect opportunity. By using colour only in your eyeliner, and not in your eye shadow, you can still create illusion whilst not drawing attention away from the eyes themselves. Suitable lively colours for use as eyeliner have been included in the colour chart (see opposite). An example of blue eyeliner used to pick up the colour of clothing and to enhance the colour of the eye can also be seen in the photograph on page 48.

Eyeliner offers the best opportunity of adding colour to an otherwise neutral palette.

eyeliner variations

Eyeliner applied all the way round the eye does not suit everyone. The size and shape of the eye will determine the most effective way of framing.

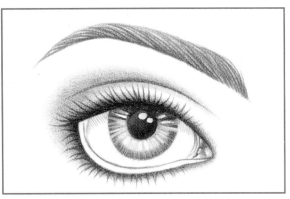

A large eye can be framed all the way round the top and bottom, using black or a dark framing colour.

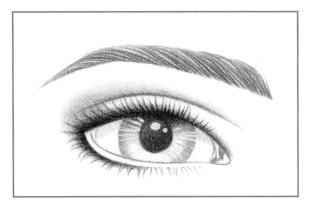

Medium and small eyes can seem smaller if they are framed all the way round. Frame the top, but only the outer section of the lower lid, if at all.

pencil eyeliner

Make sure that your eyeliner pencil has a soft and creamy consistency (see page 23), so that you are able to blend the line without stretching the skin around the eye too much. If you have just sharpened your pencil, use a tissue to round off any sharp edges. This will limit the danger of scratching the skin, and a rounded tip will give a more natural finish.

If your lashes are sparse, avoid using pencil eyeliner, as the line created will appear thick and unnatural.

liquid eyeliner

This only looks effective if you are able to create a clean, thin line. Liquid eyeliner does not suit everyone, or every occasion – ask an honest friend for her opinion. If you do decide to use this liquid, make sure that you practise the application until you have perfected the technique. In addition, obtain a high-quality liquid eyeliner brush instead of the usual applicator supplied with the product. Rest your elbow on a working surface to steady your hand.

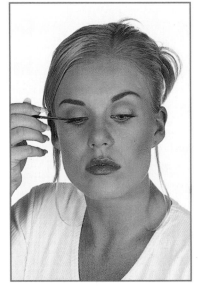

Lift your chin so that you are looking down into a mirror.

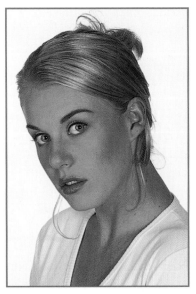

The line you apply should be thinner where it begins and ends.

mascara

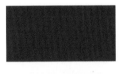

Mascara darkens and thickens the eyelashes, and makes them appear longer. Many make-up artists, myself included, only apply mascara to the top lashes for everyday make-up applications. Mascara applied to the lower lashes often smudges under the eye, and looks messy halfway through the day. The lower lashes can also create a shadow under the eye, which is accentuated by applying mascara to them. If you already have darkish rings under your eyes, this will draw attention to them. Experiment with leaving the lower lashes bare. If this feels strange and your lower lashes are very fair, it may be better to have them tinted by a beauty therapist, rather than applying mascara to them.

choosing mascara colour

Though brightly coloured eyelashes become a fashion trend from time to time (see page 87), I recommend keeping to dark brown or black mascara for everyday wear.

dark brown

black

charcoal

- ◆ for fair hair, use dark brown mascara
- ◆ for red hair, use dark brown or black mascara
- ◆ for mousy brown to black hair, use black mascara
- ◆ for grey hair, use charcoal or black mascara

> If you are using lash thickener, allow it to dry before applying mascara over it.

applying mascara

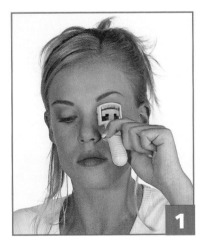

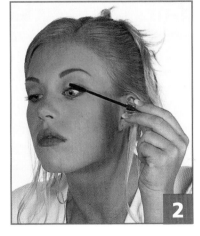

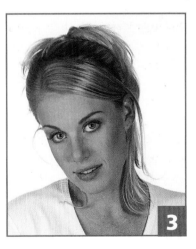

1 If you are using an eyelash curler, first curl the lashes, holding them in the curled position for 10–20 seconds.

2 Lifting your chin while looking down, stroke the mascara through your top lashes, combing them upwards.

3 To achieve a neat finish and reach the base of the lashes, use your free hand to lift the outer corner of the lid.

cheeks
get the blush

Applying make-up to her cheeks can present a woman with several tricky decisions. First and foremost, you need to decide *why* you are applying blusher to your face. Are you trying to enhance the shape of your face by contouring and creating illusions, or are you merely attempting to add some healthy-looking colour because you feel you look too pale? Both of these are valid reasons for applying blusher to your face, but they call for different choices of colour and different application techniques.

In terms of enhancing the shape of your face, blusher can be used in several ways. It can be applied in places where it serves to give more definition and prominence to cheekbones, for instance. Conversely, blusher can be used to shade and darken, or visually 'soften' cheekbones that may already be felt to be too prominent. It may also be used to create the illusion of contours that 'slim' an otherwise roundish face.

In terms of adding colour to the face, the positioning of blusher often clearly separates the amateurs from the professionals. If adding colour is your main reason for applying blusher to your cheeks, pay particular attention to the discussion on page 76.

As blusher can fulfil these two separate functions – that of contouring, and that of adding colour – one can, in fact, divide the application process into two separate stages. If your cheeks already possess natural colour, you may not need to add blusher colour to achieve a healthy-looking glow. On the other hand, if your cheekbones are already quite sharply defined, you may not need to add any form of contouring, only a little colour.

It is important, therefore, to study the shape of your face and decide *why* you are applying blusher. Then use this section to guide you in terms of *where* to apply it, and *which colours* to choose to create the particular effect you desire. In my experience most women find that they can define or contour, as well as adding colour. The first stage of the application will thus consist of using neutral colours to define the shape of your face. The second stage will involve adding colour.

Whatever your particular reason for applying blusher to your cheeks, the *art* lies in being able to position the colour in the exact area to create the desired effect, without making the blusher colour 'stripy' or obvious in any way.

blusher colours

cool

highlighters

warm

highlighters

shading colours

shading colours

choosing blusher colours

As you did when selecting eye-shadow colours, you will need to choose blusher colours from either the warm or cool palette, depending on the undertone of your skin. If you have not yet identified your undertone colour, you will need to do so now before continuing (see pages 48–55).

When faced with a blusher colour, ask yourself the following question: *can I see more pink or mauve tones in this blusher, or can I see more orange and yellow tones?* Pink and mauve tones suggest a cool colour and orange and yellow tones suggest a warm colour. If you have a cool skin undertone, select blusher from the cool colour palette. If you have a warm skin undertone, select blusher from the warm colour palette.

key

- ■ preferably for evening applications – not suitable for fair skin tones
- ❯ to add natural colour to the face after shading colours have been applied

highlighting and shading

The same principle of highlighting and shading that was used to plan the application of eye shadow will be used here. To refresh your memory, refer to pages 58 and 61. The basic rule is: *light colours bring forward and make areas appear larger or more prominent; dark colours make areas recede and look smaller or less prominent.* As you were able to create illusions using light and dark shades on your eyelids and surrounding the eyes, you will here learn how to create illusions on your cheeks.

White, cream or very light colours are called highlighters. All the other colours arranged below the highlighters in the colour charts on the previous page are called shading colours. Different effects can be achieved, depending on which part of the cheek is shaded. Look at the examples on the right.

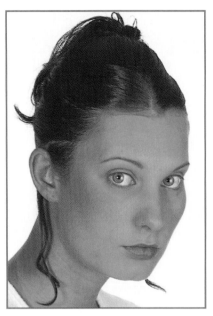

To soften a cheekbone that may already be quite prominent, the shading colour is applied along the bone itself.

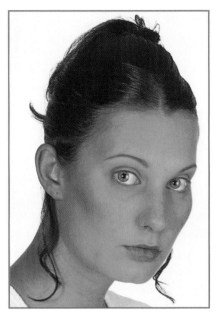

To add definition to the cheekbone or to slim the face, the shading colour is applied in a curved shape below the cheekbone.

softening a prominent cheekbone

If you feel that your cheekbones are too 'sharp' and prominent, you can 'soften' them by referring to the illustration below, and by following the steps outlined.

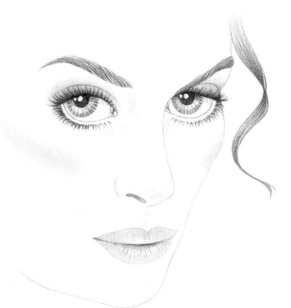

1 Simply apply a suitable shading colour (cool or warm neutral) along the cheekbone itself, as shown in the illustration on the left. This will darken the bone area, and create the illusion of it being less prominent.

2 Using a slightly larger brush, blend the colour well so that there is no hard, definite 'stripe' of colour along the cheekbone. Blending is essential to achieving a professional-looking finish.

defining a cheekbone or slimming a face

To give more definition to the cheekbone, or to slim the face, refer to the illustration below, and follow the steps outlined. The photographs refer to step 1 and step 2 only.

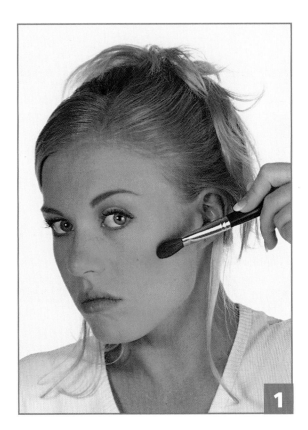

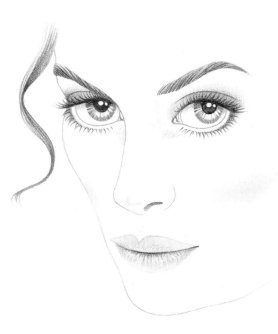

Shading is applied in a curved shape below the bone.

1 Apply a shading colour below the cheekbone, using a small, dome-shaped blusher brush.

2 Apply highlighter along the bone itself, using a slightly larger brush.

3 Now blend the 'edges' of the colours well using a clean brush. There should be no distinguishable 'bands' of colour and the presence of blusher should not be obvious in any way.

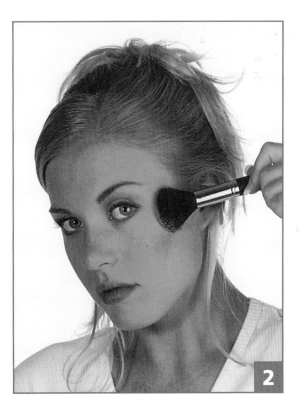

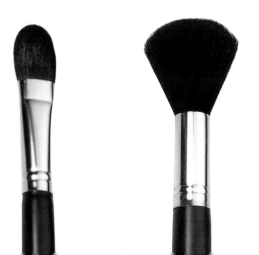

adding colour

'Colour' can be added to the face after contouring (highlighting and shading) has taken place. The best colour to choose is a very natural soft pink (marked with a ◗ in the colour chart on page 73). The pink colour should not stand out as an 'added' colour, but should look like a natural glow – as if you had just pinched your cheeks.

The colour on the immediate right is a natural pink blush, whereas the colour further to the right is too bright a pink to look natural.

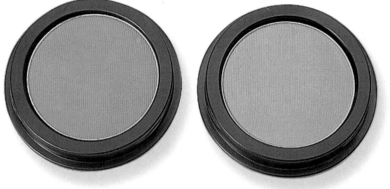

Even if you have a warm skin undertone, use a natural pink colour, as everyone goes a little pink when warm or excited. Do not think that you have to add bright orange to your cheeks to brighten your face if you have a warm skin undertone. You will, however, still be using a colour with a warm tone to it to contour your face.

If you want to add healthy-looking colour to your face – in addition to contouring – refer to the illustration and the photograph below.

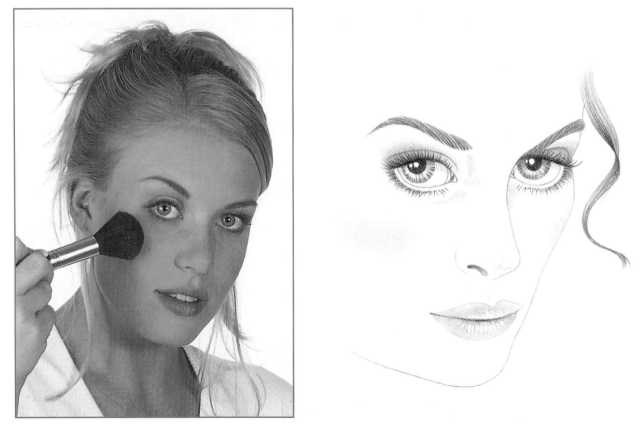

A very natural pink colour should be lightly dusted onto the cheek in the position indicated on the illustration.

the importance of positioning blusher correctly

Although the cheekbone does not slant downwards across the face in a straight line, many women apply their blusher in a straight line or 'band'. If you apply light pressure, and feel along your cheekbone, you will realize that it curves up slightly towards the front of the face. If you are applying shading colour to enhance the bone, the colour should therefore also be applied in a slight curve along the lower side of the bone, and below it.

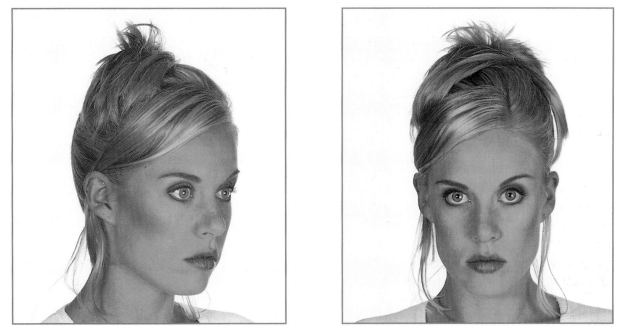

This side and front view of the same application illustrates how the contouring blusher shade correctly enhances the shape of the bone by following its natural curved shape.

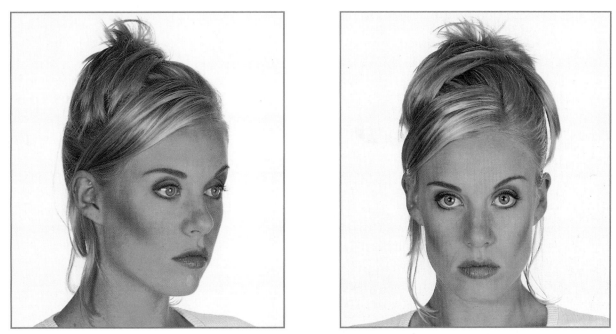

This side and front view of the same application shows how the contouring blusher shade has been incorrectly applied in a straight line. Note how the colour finishes too low towards the front of the face. It drags the shape of the face downwards and creates a 'hard' look.

lips
get the colour

Lipstick adds the finishing touch to a look by defining the mouth and adding colour to the face. It is also the step during which you can have the most fun, as there are fewer make-up 'rules' and restrictions here than anywhere else. You can transform your look in any way you like, simply by changing your lipstick colour. In a matter of seconds you can go from next-to-natural, to casual, elegant, dramatic or fun and funky. And by mixing lipsticks on the lips you can create your own unique colours.

Remember, however, that lipstick applied by itself to a face otherwise bare of make-up, will usually draw attention to any blemishes, redness or unevenness in skin tone. Examples of this effect can clearly be seen in the photographs used on pages 50 and 51. If you are applying lipstick, therefore, or changing the natural colour of your lips in any way, always ensure that your overall look is balanced. Apply foundation to even out your skin tone, and add other make-up products as well to complete your look.

decisions, decisions

Most women have the luxury of owning a variety of lipstick colours, and of being able to select a particular colour to suit a particular occasion. Your choice of colour usually depends on several factors. Firstly, you will have to determine whether you have a cool or warm skin tone, and select all your lipstick colours from either the cool or the warm palette. This is discussed in detail on pages 49–55.

Secondly, your choice of lipstick colour will be determined to some extent by the colours of the clothing you are wearing. Your lipstick colour should not clash with your outfit, for example, but complement it. If you are wearing a smart red blazer for a business meeting, for instance, an application of an equally strong red lipstick can be highly effective and communicate your confidence.

The last factor to consider is the style of dress, in terms of casual daily wear or smart evening attire. If you are wearing casual jeans and a T-shirt, I would recommend a natural lip colour rather than a deep burgundy, for instance. On the other hand, if you are wearing an evening gown, strong, dark lip colours may be preferable to pale peach or pearly pink. Refer to the photographs of the glamorous evening look created on page 67, for example, or to the section on fun and funky looks for the young on pages 86–87.

lipstick colours

Many make-up houses do not separate their cool and warm colours for display purposes, so you will have to use your own judgement to categorize a lipstick as either cool or warm. (Cool and warm colours are discussed in detail on pages 48–57.)

Before purchasing lipstick, test the colour on the back of your hand. Ask yourself whether you can see more pink or mauve tones in the colour, or whether you can see more orange and yellow tones. If you see more pink or mauve tones, the colour is cool; if you can see more orange or yellow tones, it is a warm colour.

The lipstick colour chart reproduced on page 80 illustrates just some of the many colours I would recommend, both from the cool and the warm palette.

applying make-up to the lips

There are several products and several techniques involved in applying make-up to the lips in a professional way. It is important to know why and how each product is used, and why, when and how certain techniques are applied. Treat your lips well, as chapped, dry or flaky lips can be a nightmare to work with.

moisturizing dry lips

If your lips are dry, first soften them by applying a lip balm and allowing it a few minutes to soak into the skin. Then blot the lips on a tissue to remove excess oiliness.

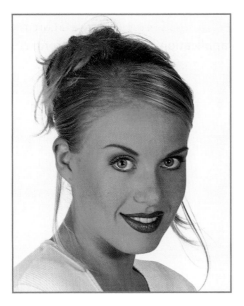

If you have been brave enough to buy a very different colour to what you are used to wearing, experiment over weekends. Apply the lip colour while you are at home, and look at yourself in the mirror every now and again. By doing this, you will gradually 'train' your eye to like it.

Your lipstick application technique can 'make or break' your look. Whether you opt for a natural or dark lipstick colour, aim to achieve a balanced overall effect.

techniques

cool

warm

choosing lipstick colours

Once you have narrowed down your selection of colours, *try them on your lips* to test the colour properly. The same lipstick used by a friend may well produce a different colour on your own lips. You may need to go out of the store to check the colour in natural light, as fluorescent light can distort your perception of the true colour.

The colours reproduced on this page are only a small selection of the endless variety available. They are intended merely as a guide to either the cool or the warm shades that may suit you. If you struggle to choose colours when faced with the array at the cosmetics counter, you may want to take this book along to guide you.

key

+ not recommended for small lips

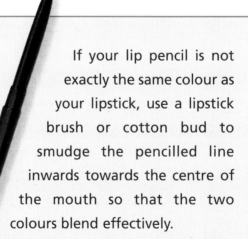

If your lip pencil is not exactly the same colour as your lipstick, use a lipstick brush or cotton bud to smudge the pencilled line inwards towards the centre of the mouth so that the two colours blend effectively.

lining the lips

Use a lip pencil in the same colour as the lipstick or in a slightly darker colour. The qualities of a good lip pencil are discussed on page 24. The pencil should be sharpened and any scratchy edges can then be softened slightly on a tissue.

When lining your lips, do not simply start along the upper lip and work you way round the mouth, following the natural lip edge. If you want to correct any 'faults' in terms of lip shape – and very few people have perfectly symmetrical mouths – it will be easier to do on a mouth bare of colour. The easiest way to balance the appearance of your lips whilst lining, is to divide the mouth into sections, and work on each part in turn until the lines are connected.

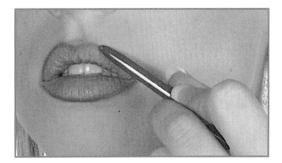

Follow the numbering in the illustration below – and the corresponding text – to learn the correct sequence when pencilling.

1 Start in the middle of the upper lip, and line the Cupid's bow as shown. You will immediately be able to see where other sections of your lips may be uneven.

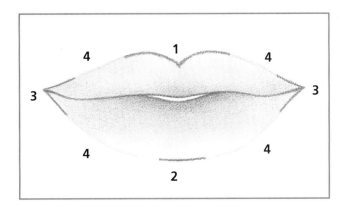

2 Now move to the centre of your bottom lip, and draw a short, horizontal line.

3 The next step is to line the corners of your mouth. If your lips are asymmetric, refer to the illustration at the bottom of this page. If your lips are close to symmetrical, carefully draw in two neat corners.

4 Finally, connect the lines drawn in the centre (top and bottom) to the corners.

correcting the lip shape

If your lips are irregular or asymmetric in shape, as illustrated below, it is possible to create the illusion of almost perfectly balanced lips when lining your lips with pencil.

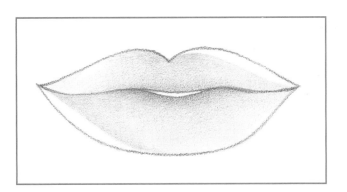

1 Follow the same sequence set out above for lining uneven lips. Line the centres of your lips first, before moving to the corners.

2 Create the illusion of balance between your top and bottom lips by 'correcting' your lip shape subtly, ensuring that your pencilled lines meet precisely at the corners. In this example, both the upper and lower lips have been 'corrected' in terms of shape.

applying lipstick

1 Use a small, firm lipstick brush of sable hair (see page 13) to apply lipstick. Work carefully, creating a smooth, clean edge. If you apply lipstick straight from the tube, you will never achieve a perfect edge, and you will need to re-apply lipstick more frequently.

2 Blot your lips on a tissue and apply a second coat.

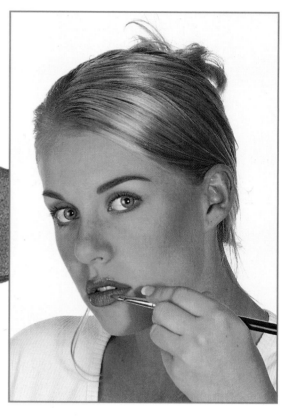

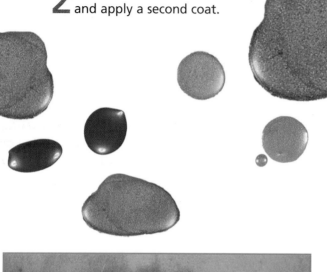

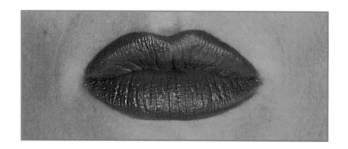

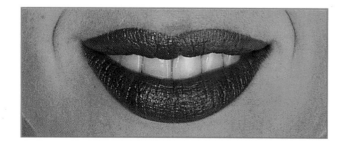

practice makes perfect

Take great care when applying lipstick in dark colours, as any of the following common mistakes will be more obvious.

Left: *Avoid irregular lip edges like these, which look really messy.*

Left: *Take care not to work too far out beyond the natural edge. This will only make it obvious that you would prefer having fuller lips. Also refer to page 81, in terms of 'correcting' the lip shape.*

Left: *Edges should be clean and neat, following the natural lip line as closely as possible.*

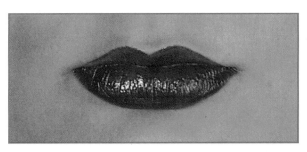

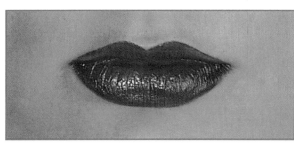

Here a smaller top lip has been filled in incorrectly, and the corners do not look balanced (refer to the discussion of asymmetric lips on page 81).

The corners of the top lip have now been correctly filled out to meet those of the bottom lip, creating an illusion of balance. The look is still perfectly natural.

applying lip gloss

Lips high on gloss tend to come and go as a make-up trend, so keep an eye on the fashions of the time. Lip gloss is applied after lipstick, and then only to the centre of lips. Applied close to the edge of your lips, lip gloss tends to 'bleed' beyond the lip edges. If your lipstick tends to bleed in any case, avoid adding lip gloss. Mature skins, especially, should avoid using lip gloss.

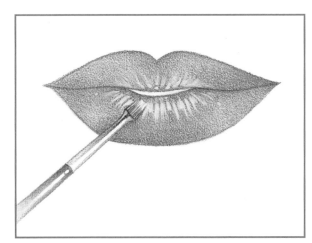

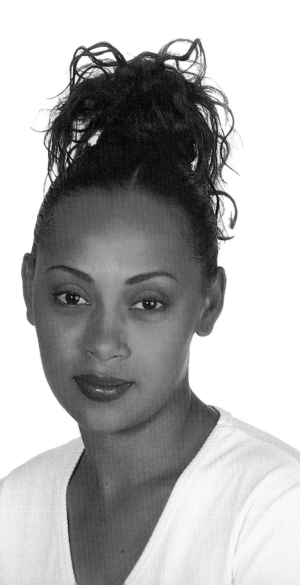

Above and right: *Apply lip gloss to the centre of the lips only, to avoid lipstick bleeding beyond the edges of the lip line. Here lip gloss is also used to enhance attractive, full lips.*

colour that lasts

If you want your lipstick application to last as long as possible without re-application being necessary, I recommend using matte lipstick. Several layers of lipstick can be applied, and lips should be blotted on a tissue before each new layer is applied.

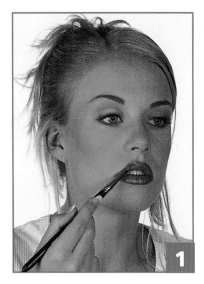

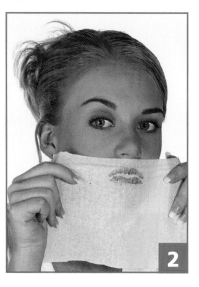

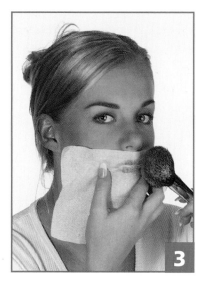

1 Apply matte lipstick, which usually lasts longer than any other kind.

2 After applying one layer of lipstick, gently blot the lips on a tissue.

3 Then apply a light dusting of loose powder through the tissue.

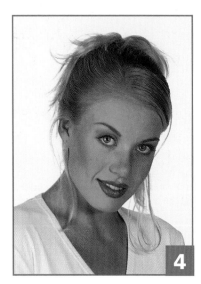

4 Apply a final layer of lipstick, but do not apply powder over it.

Unfortunately, the longer you want your lipstick to last, the dryer the lipstick has to be, and this can begin to feel uncomfortable. A creamier lipstick will keep your lips softer, but, owing to the added moisture in the lipstick, it will not last as long. There is no happy medium here. If you want lip colour that lasts, you have to sacrifice the comfort of soft lips. If you want soft, comfortable lips, you will have to sacrifice staying power.

mature skin

As one ages, your colouring in terms of skin, lips, eyes and hair changes subtly. This means that colours that may have looked great on your face at twenty, may no longer be flattering at thirty or forty. The colours may be too strong for your skin tone or too pale to add colour to a face that needs more brightening than it used to.

When it comes to choosing lipstick colours, pale, frosted or pearly shades should be avoided completely. These are the least flattering on mature skin. Also avoid lip gloss.

The most common problem in the case of mature skin, is that of lipstick 'bleeding' or spreading outwards from the lips into the fine lines around the mouth. To help prevent this, follow the steps outlined below, and study the photographs.

1 Use a high-quality lip pencil – not soft and smudgy – to neatly define the outline of your lips. In addition to lining the lips, also use the pencil to shade the lips lightly.

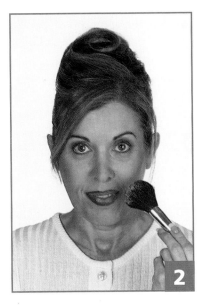

2 Apply loose powder to the entire shaded area, and then apply a *matte* lipstick. (These lipsticks are drier and less creamy and will therefore not bleed as easily).

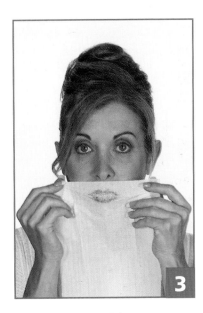

3 Gently press the lips onto a tissue to blot.

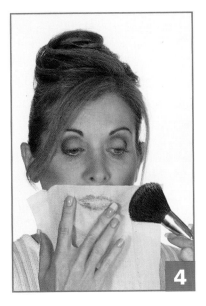

4 Lightly dust loose powder onto the lips through the tissue, using a powder brush.

5 Repeat the process set out here two to three times, finishing with an application of loose powder.

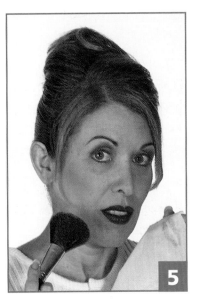

over the top
and funky just for fun

There is always a time and a place just for having fun – and where almost no make-up 'rules' apply. An adventurous night on the town provides a perfect opportunity to delight your fancy in the latest fashion fads. Add sparkle and colour – the more the better. Shine and shimmer to your heart's content. Wow the crowds who go clubbing and outshine the dance floor's lights!

breaking all the rules

As many regular clubbers will agree, half the fun of the party lies in planning and preparing your look. The other half is enjoying showing off what you have accomplished. Now is the time to break all the rules, and make use of the enormous variety of fun products. And make-up application is certainly not limited to the face alone – use it on shoulders, collarbones, and even on your hair. Body paint is fun and funky, and you can keep everyone guessing by applying a little temporary 'tattoo' in the form of a cheeky transfer or stencilled shape.

shimmer dust or glitter dust is a loose, fine eye-shadow powder with a high shimmer or sparkle content that 'lights up' as light strikes it. The powder colour will determine its positioning. Gold and pearl can be dusted virtually anywhere; pinks and mauves are great for cheeks or eyes, but green and blue are best kept for the eyes. Use a brush, tapping off excess powder onto a tissue, and lightly dust only a small amount of powder on at a time.

a pearlized finish can be achieved by using a pearlized foundation or cream in stick form. This can be applied lightly over the entire face – and body – using a latex sponge. It is very effective to highlight specific areas like cheekbones and browbones.

glitter gel is one of the easiest and quickest ways of transforming any look to suit the club. It can be used anywhere on the face or body, over or without other make-up products, and it is available in a variety of colours. Usually one finds a clear gel base, carrying coloured glitter. Coloured glitter gel consists of a *coloured* gel base carrying glitter. This provides instant colour as well as glitter – a wonderful substitute for eye shadow.

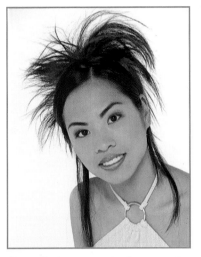

Here dark green shadow creates evening eyes. Lips are kept quite natural, only given a pearly finish.

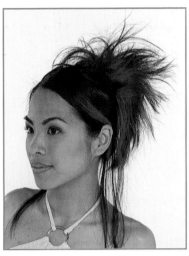

Gold dust highlights brows and cheekbones. Blue and green face paint make for 'mermaid' lips.

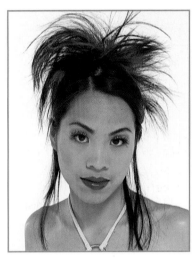

Go over the top with false lashes in metallic green. Strengthen .the mouth with plummy lip gloss.

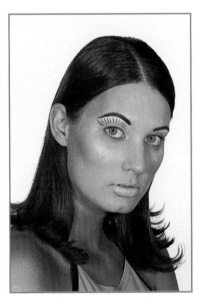

face paint or eye paint can be used to add bold, fun colours and dramatic painted shapes. Seen under flashing lights, the effect is striking. Icy pastel shades combine well with strong colours.

brightly coloured hair can easily be achieved using coloured hair mascara or spray. Use fluorescent colours on very dark hair, and almost anything but gold on blonde hair – then simply wash the colour out.

stick-on shapes can be applied by just using a little petroleum jelly as an adhesive. Add a few stars to a cheek or temple, or develop your own design.

use colour when and wherever you like – there are no limits. Go green on eyes, as shown at the top of this page. Or outline lips in intense purple, using a cotton bud to blend the edges inwards. Keep centres of lips more natural, adding just a touch of glitter.

literally, almost anything goes . . .

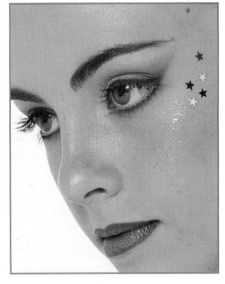

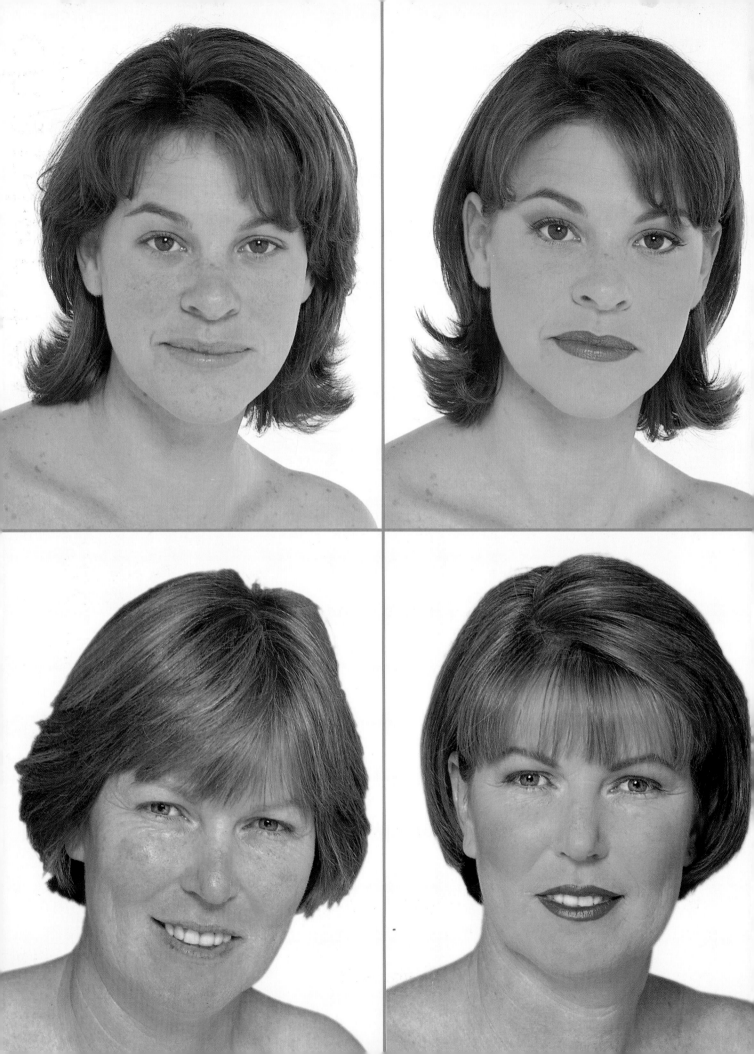

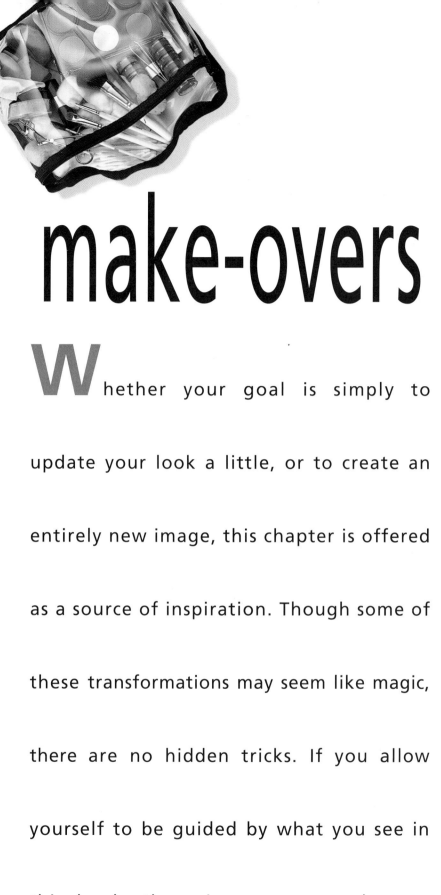

make-overs

Whether your goal is simply to update your look a little, or to create an entirely new image, this chapter is offered as a source of inspiration. Though some of these transformations may seem like magic, there are no hidden tricks. If you allow yourself to be guided by what you see in this book, there is no reason why you cannot create looks like these yourself.

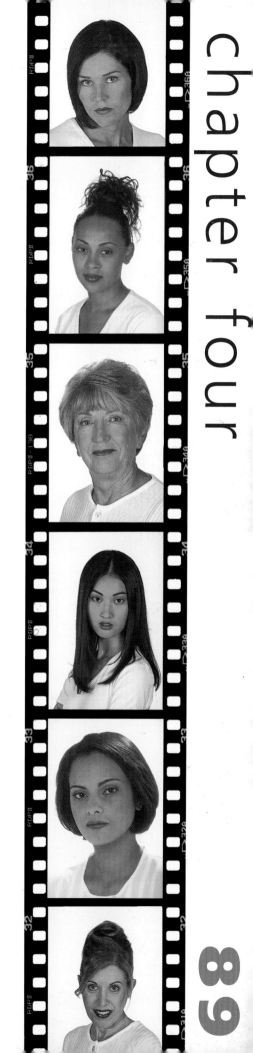

make-overs
make magic

During my career as a professional make-up artist and teacher, scores of women have consulted me about changing and enhancing their looks. All too often, though, before I have had a chance to say anything, they have also already told me what kind of look they *do not* want.

It is a fact that we all grow used to and comfortable with seeing ourselves looking a particular way. We react with shock when we suddenly see our comfortable image having been altered by a hairstylist, for instance. Or we balk at the mere suggestion of trying something altogether different. We feel that we know ourselves better than anyone else, and are therefore able to judge better than anyone else what suits us and what does not.

The truth is that we are very rarely able to look at ourselves objectively. It is important, therefore, when considering a change, not to defend against suggestions immediately. If you are consulting a professionally trained make-up artist or hairstylist, listen carefully to their ideas. Their advice will be based on their professional opinion – informed by their training, expertise and experience.

Practise using your judgement by studying the two photographs on this page, and deciding which make-up application enhances the face most, creating a younger, fresher appearance.

which is better?

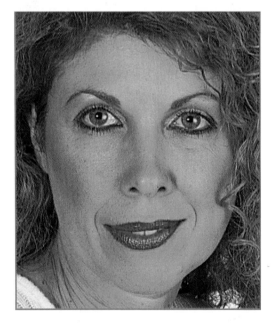
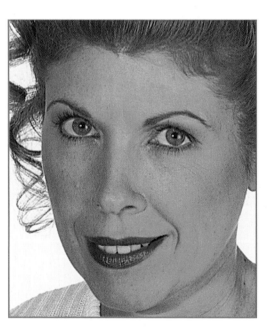

shimmer eye shadow?
coloured products, like eye shadow?
dark, pencilled eyeliner?
hard, strong blusher?
glossy lipstick?

or

subtle, matte eye shadow?
neutral eye shadow and other products?
smoky, blended shadow as eyeliner?
soft, natural blusher?
matte lipstick?

making the change & sticking with it

Even if you feel uncomfortable with a new look at first and immediately want to revert to what you are used to, decide to give your new image a chance. Do not restyle your hair or wash off all your make-up the minute you reach home. Ask yourself whether you really know what suits you best, or whether you just know what you have become used to. After a few weeks of 'bearing with' your new style of make-up or haircut, you may find yourself wondering why you did not change before.

The information provided in this book gives you the key to looking great – anywhere, and anytime. No matter what your colouring, your age or your lifestyle – you will always look your best in 'nearly natural', neutral, matte make-up. Look at the variety of women included in this chapter.

I sincerely hope that this series of make-overs inspires you to use the art of make-up to make the most of yourself – always.

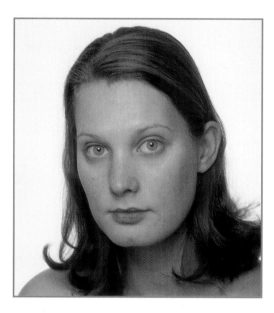

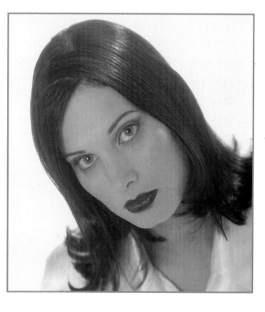

before

after

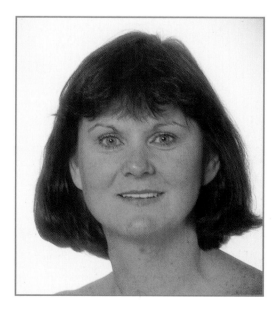

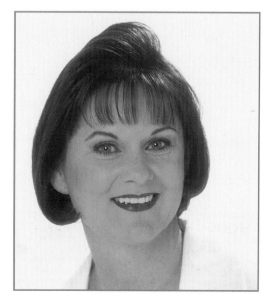

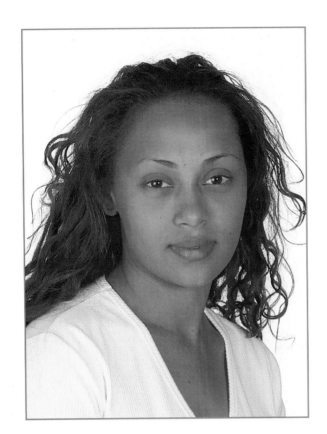

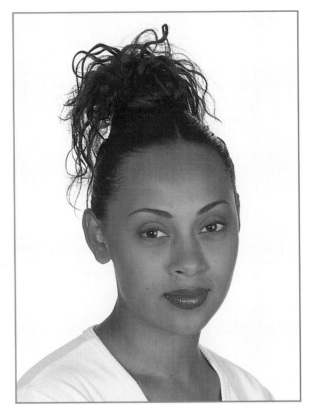

before

after

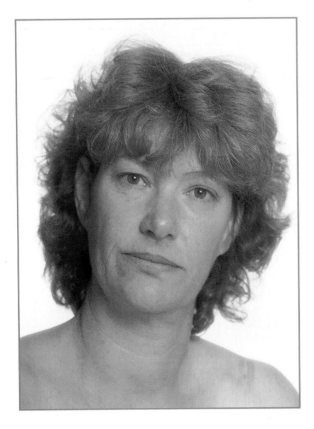

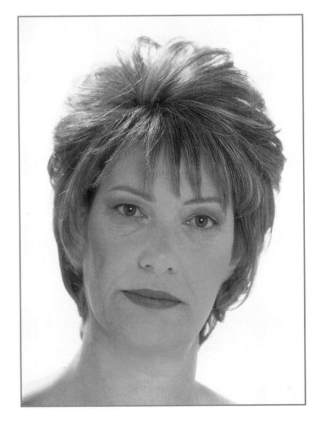

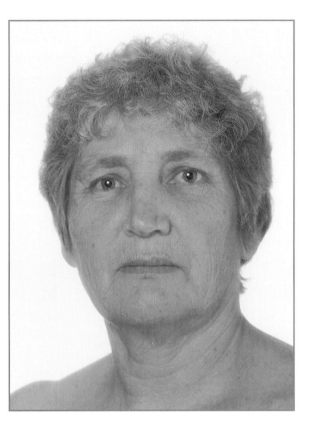

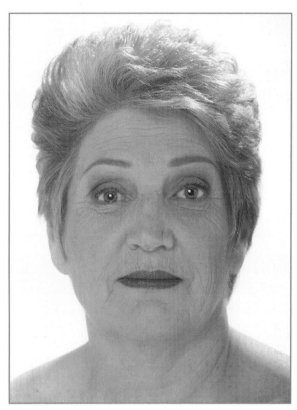

before   after

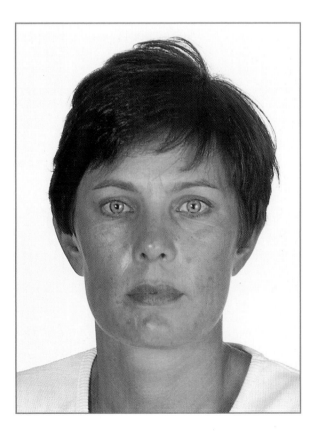

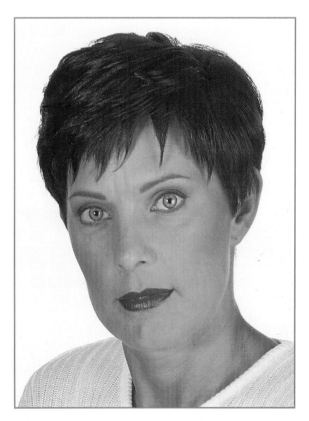

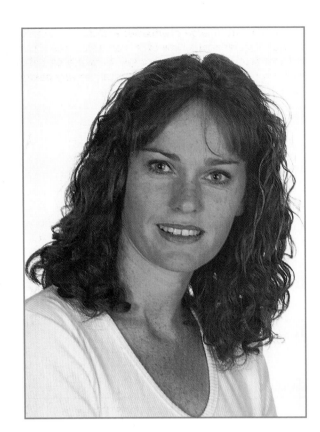

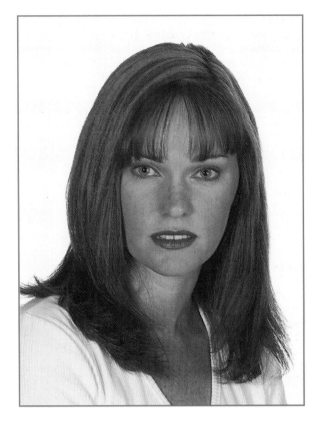

before

after

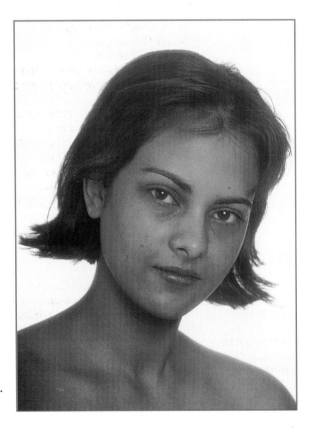

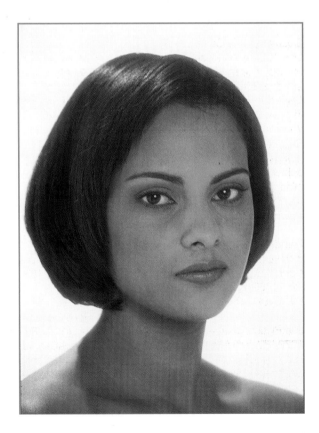

Most of the products and equipment discussed in this book are available from large pharmacies and department stores with good cosmetics counters. Some readers who may not live near a major centre, however, may experience difficulty in obtaining certain items. These readers are encouraged to contact a professional supplier closest to their area, selected from the list provided below. These suppliers do not deal only with professional make-up artist but can be very helpful to anyone seriously interested in the art of make-up, or in obtaining a particular product or accessory.

Alcone Co
549 49th Avenue
Long Island City
NY 11101-5610, USA
Tel: (718) 361 8373
Mail-order suppliers for make-up of all brands.

California Theatrical Supply
132 9th Street
San Francisco
CA 94103-2603, USA
Tel: (415) 863 923
Distributors of Kryolan make-up to the West Coast of the USA.

Charles H Fox Ltd
22 Tavistock Street, Covent Garden
London WC2E 7PY
England
Tel: (020) 7240 3111

Cinema Secrets
4400 West Riverside Drive
Burbank
CA 91505-4097, USA
Tel: (818) 563 9213
Suppliers of a full line of professional make-up products.

Cosmetics a la Carte Ltd
Unit 102, Avro House
Havelock Terrace
London SW8 4AS
England
Tel/Fax: (020) 7622 2318
Website: www.a-la-carte.co.uk
Suppliers of a full line of professional make-up, specializing in hard-to-find colours. Free brochure and full mail-order service of products and equipment, as well as a studio to visit for individual lessons or practical advice.

Frends Beauty Supply Co
5270 Laurel Canyon Boulevard
North Hollywood
CA 91607-2792, USA
Tel: (818) 769 3834

Joe Blasco, Cosmetics
1670 Hillhurst Ave # 202-3
Los Angeles
CA 90027-5580, USA
Suppliers of the full Joe Blasco Cosmetic line.

Kryolan Corp
132 9th Street
San Francisco
CA 94103-2603
USA
Tel: (415) 863 9236
Suppliers of a full line of theatrical make-up.

Make-up Center Ltd
150 West 55th Street
New York City
NY 10019-5305
USA
Tel: (212) 997 9494

Make Up For Ever
Hyde Park Corner
Jan Smuts Avenue
Johannesburg
South Africa
Tel: (011) 325 5035

Josie Knowland
Film Make Up Technology
5 The Crescent
Annandale
NSW 2038
Australia
Tel: (02) 9518 9000

Make Up For Ever
Sandton City Shopping Centre
Sandton
Johannesburg
South Africa
Tel: (011) 883 7091

The Make-up School (Cape Town)
P.O. Box 6672
Welgemoed
7538
South Africa
Tel: (021) 910 4150

The Make-up School (Johannesburg)
P.O. Box 1877
Rivonia
2128
South Africa
Tel: (011) 807 2844
Full nationwide mail-order service for products and equipment, as well as professional training and individual make-up classes.

Naimie's Beauty Center
12640 Riverside Drive
North Hollywood
CA 91607-3411, USA
Tel: (818) 655 9933
Fax: (818) 655 9999
Website: www.naimies.com
Professional suppliers of over 50 different brands of make-up and accessories.

Professional Make-up
Cavendish Square
Cavendish Street
Claremont
South Africa
Tel: (021) 671 3344

Professional Make-up
Tyger Valley Centre
Willie van Schoor Avenue
Bellville, South Africa
Tel: (021) 914 3410

Screenface
24 Powis Terrace, London
W11 1JH, England
Tel: (020) 7221 8289
and
48 Monmouth Street, London
WC2H 9EP, England
Tel: (020) 7836 3955
Suppliers of a full line of all professional make-up products and accessories.

There are now various salons throughout South Africa that stock Professional Make-up products. As these details constantly change (salons move or new salons arise), we have introduced an information line whereby readers from all over the country can call to enquire about a stockist in their area. For more information, please call (0860) 10 21 25.

To obtain further information on the availability of quality make-up tools or products, write to the author:

Joy Terri
P.O. Box 6672
Welgemoed
7538
South Africa